WHAT'S REALLY
IN OUR FOOD?
Fact and Fiction
About Fat and Fiber,
Vitamins and Minerals,
Nutrients and Contaminants

WHAT'S REALLY IN OUR FOOD?

Fact and Fiction About Fat and Fiber, Vitamins and Minerals, Nutrients and Contaminants

Mia Parsonnet, M.D.

Illustrated by Kathy Cadow Parsonnet

SHAPOLSKY PUBLISHERS, Inc.
New York

A Shapolsky Book

For any additional information, contact:
Shapolsky Publishers, Inc.
126 West 22nd Street
New York, NY 10011
(212) 633-2022
FAX (212) 633-2123

10 9 8 7 6 5 4 3 2 1

Library of Congress Cataloging-in-Publication Data
Parsonnet, Mia.
      What's Really in Our Food? Fact and fiction about fat
      and fiber, vitamins and minerals, nutrients and
      contaminants/Mia Parsonnet.
      ISBN 1-56171-034-2 (softcover)
      1. Nutrition. I. Title
QP141.P345   1991
613.2—dc20   91-9055

Design by Sherrel Farnsworth
Typography by Smith Inc.
Manufactured in the United States of America

ACKNOWLEDGMENTS

I want to thank my husband, Dr. Victor Parsonnet, for his patience and invaluable help and support; and Dr. Julie Parsonnet, Dr. Muriel Fox, and Dr. Gertrude Sobel for their thoughtful suggestions during the preparation of this manuscript.

Mia Parsonnet, M.D.
Millburn, New Jersey
1991

CONTENTS

Introduction

We are constantly bombarded by ads that tell us what is good for us and what we shouldn't do without. But which of these claims is true, and which is double-talk? What do we really need in our daily diet, and how do we get it?

Many of us know more about the mix we feed our African violets and the gasoline we put in our cars than about the food we eat. We look at phosphorus and nitrogen in plant food, and at octanes and additives in gas, and hope that this attention will keep the flowers blooming and the engines humming. When it comes to ourselves, however, we tend to be less well informed, perhaps in the mistaken belief that the body will take care of itself.

Our ideas about nutrution are changing constantly. There are no guarantees that what we know today will not be discredited tomorrow, or, on the other hand, that some far-out claims won't ultimately prove their worth. Still, the field of nutrition has a solid base, enhanced in recent years by a huge amount of interest and study.

This book is intended to provide basic information to the consumer about all the substances we eat. I have made an effort to present as fact what is fact, to identify conjectures and fads, and to demystify some terms and concepts that have become part of our vocabulary, whether we quite understand them or not.

CHAPTER I

Building Blocks

The human organism is the most complex entity we know. Nothing could be more intricate in structure and function. The uniqueness of living things is linked primarily to proteins, substances that are produced *only* by living cells, and without which life cannot exist.

PROTEIN

Protein molecules are large and complex. They consist of long chains of amino acids, the protein "building blocks." The type, number and arrangement of amino acids characterizes each of the myriads of different proteins.

After a protein meal the body splits these large molecules into amino acids and fashions them to form new proteins, characteristic of the species. Animal proteins contain a more favorable assortment of amino acids for our diet, but vegetarians can attain good nutrition by choosing their foods judiciously. Soybeans provide one of the best vegetable proteins. The cultivation of soybeans was started in ancient times in China, but the United States now grows more soybeans than any other country.

Adequate protein intake is essential for growth and bodily

functioning. Young children require a minimum of an ounce of pure protein daily. For non-pregnant adults the amount is about 2 ounces. This sounds like very little, but, with the exception of egg whites, foods do not consist of pure protein. It takes about 3 or 4 ounces of meat or fish, or a quart of milk, or 5 eggs to provide just one ounce (28 gm) of protein. The same amount, though not the same quality of protein can also be obtained from 4 cups of cooked spaghetti or 2½ cups of cooked lima beans.

The healthy body tries to preserve protein; protein is utilized for fuel only when carbohydrate and fat stores have been depleted, such as occurs in starvation. Proteins and fats can be made into carbohydrates and be used for energy; proteins and carbohydrates can be converted to fat and be deposited as such; but neither fats nor carbohydrates can create proteins.

AMINO ACIDS

Good nutrition depends to a great extent on the quality of the protein we eat. Proteins are composed of amino acids; the characteristics and nutritional value of a protein are determined by the arrangement and type of its constituent amino acids. Amino acids are also the building blocks of hormones and enzymes.

In human beings about two dozen amino acids are necessary for good nutrition. Nine of them are called "essential." This does not mean that they contribute more to nutrition than non-essential ones; it simply means that they must be taken in the diet because the human body is unable to manufacture them from more basic food stuffs or from other amino acids (with two limited exceptions, listed below).

For maximum nutritional benefit, a proper assortment of amino acids must be available at the same time. Animal proteins, such as are found in meat, fish, eggs and dairy products, provide not only a greater concentration, but also a greater variety of essential amino acids than vegetable proteins. Nevertheless, by being informed and selecting proper *combinations* of vegetable products, vegetarians can achieve good protein nutrition. Rice and red beans or rice and lentils, for example, are good sources, as are chickpeas and sesame seeds, or beans and cheese. All of these combinations are common in different parts of the world, reflecting a bit of folk wisdom. The greatest potential hazard for strict vegetarians is a deficiency in Vitamin B_{12}.

The essential amino acids are: histidine, isoleucine, leucine, lysine, methionine, (cystine can substitute in part), phenylalanine (tyrosine can substitute in part), threonine, tryptophan and valine. Arginine is sometimes included in this list. It can be synthesized, but not always in sufficient quantities during maximum growth periods. Extra amounts may also be needed when there is unusual stress, such as with surgery or serious illness.

The actual quantities needed of each amino acid are quite small. If all the essential amino acids were lumped together in pure form, they would add up to a quarter of an ounce per day for an average person.

Except on very restricted diets (eating only one or two foods), deficiency of a single amino acid does not occur. Supplements are not recommended; they are expensive, and may actually upset the desirable amino acid balance. Amino acid supplements have been touted to athletes as muscle builders. The best that can be said for them in this regard is that they are probably less harmful than anabolic steroids. Long term effects of large doses are not yet known.

Two amino acids have received some special attention recently: tryptophan, because it is a precursor of serotonin, is reputed to have a calming effect; and tyrosine, because it is a precursor of adrenaline, is said to act as a stimulant, increasing alertness and memory. Tryptophan has not proved itself in this regard, and serious side effects have been reported (possibly due to a contaminant). Tyrosine is being tested in patients who suffer attacks of irresistible sleep (narcolepsy), but there is no evidence that it acts as an energizer in healthy people.

PURINES

In the body, purines are normal breakdown-products of certain proteins. In some medical conditions—particularly in gout—purine metabolism is disturbed, and one of the purines, uric acid, rises in the blood and may be deposited in the joints, causing painful attacks of arthritis. In gout and several other diseases, foods with a high purine yield should be avoided.

Foods Highest in Purines

ORGAN MEATS	Sweetbreads, liver, kidneys, brains
SEAFOOD	Anchovies, sardines, herring, scallops
MEAT	All meats and meat extracts

Foods Lowest in Purines

Fruits and nuts
Dairy products
Eggs
Refined cereals and breads
Coffee and tea

FASCINATING FACTS ABOUT PROTEINS

- Brown eggs have the same nutritional value as white eggs.

- Raw or undercooked meat, poultry, and raw fish carry some risk of serious illness. The same is true of raw or undercooked eggs. The greatest risk comes form raw oysters and clams.

- Red meat from free-grazing animals is leaner and tougher than the meat of domestic animals. It may also be healthier, because it has a more favorable ratio of different saturated fatty acids. That means that venison, buffalo or goat meat is less likely to raise blood cholesterol than ranch raised beef.

- Surplus protein in the diet is burned for energy or stored as fat. It does not add to muscle tissue or increase muscle power. The way to enlarge and strengthen muscles is to exercise them.

- A high-protein diet usually includes a lot of fat. In fact, some high-protein foods (like a fine steak) get more calories from fat than from protein. In a so-called healthy breakfast of orange juice, bacon and eggs, buttered toast, and a glass of milk, fat provides about 53 percent of the calories, to only 15 percent of protein and 32 percent carbohydrate.

Not many years ago high-protein diets were advocated, just as complex carbohydrates are today.

CHAPTER II

Carbohydrates, Complex and Otherwise

Carbohydrates are the most abundant source of food energy, and, for most people, provide the largest part of the diet. Ideally they should constitute about 55 percent of the caloric intake, with proteins supplying 15 percent and fats 30 percent. There are three basic groups: sugars or "simple carbohydrates," starches or "complex carbohydrates," and cellulose (fiber).

The best known *sugars* are fructose (fruit sugar), sucrose (cane or beet sugar), and lactose (milk sugar), but there are several others. *Starches* are derived chiefly from cereal grains, but most vegetables and fruits consist of starches. The third group, *cellulose,* is not digested by humans; it is the fibrous part of most plant foods we eat, and provides useful roughage (and no calories). Carbohydrates are more rapidly utilized than fats or proteins, and thus supply the quickest energy; this is particularly true of sugars, which tend to provide a fast, but short-lived boost. Ultimately, most absorbed carbohydrates are broken down into the simplest of the sugars, glucose. This is the molecule that is carried in the blood stream for use by the various organs and tissues, there to be burned for energy, or to undergo another transformation that makes it suitable for storage.

Even the most restricted diet should include carbohydrates, because, aside from their own intrinsic nutritional value, they also aid in the orderly utilization of proteins and fats.

SUGAR AND OTHER CALORIC SWEETENERS

Honey bees were kept by the Egyptians more than 4,500 years ago. Sugar cane was described more than 2,000 years ago. It seems that man has always had a sweet tooth and we have never lost it. Each of us eats about 125 pounds of sugar a year.

Sugars provide calories (food energy), but virtually nothing in the way of vitamins or minerals. Since about a quarter of our daily calories are supplied by sugar (most of it in processed food), the rest of our diet had better be nutritious! We must recognize that sugar represents "empty calories," and that it also contributes to tooth decay. It does not, however, cause criminal behavior, hyperactivity, or diabetes (even though diabetes is a disease in which the blood sugar level may be high).

Table sugar provides 4 calories per gram, or 113 calories per ounce. It has less than half the calories of an equal weight of fat.

Sucrose is the most common variety and serves as our table sugar. It is obtained from sugar cane or sugar beets, and is marketed in granulated, powdered, or cube form. Sucrose is a disaccharide or double sugar, a composite of two simple sugars, glucose and fructose. In the course of digestion, sucrose is broken down into these two components.

Invert sugar also consists of glucose and fructose, but is obtained by a chemical process that splits sucrose. It is marketed in liquid form, and is used chiefly in commercial food production to maintain freshness.

Glucose is the main form of sugar normally carried in the blood stream. It supplies fuel to cells and tissues. The same formula is produced commercially from corn starch, and is known as *corn sugar* and *dextrose*.

Fructose, or fruit sugar, is found in honey and in sweet fruits. It is the sweetest of sugars, providing 1½ times as much sweetness as table sugar. The commercial form is known as *levulose*. Fructose is absorbed more slowly than sucrose and thus is less likely to produce sugar highs and lows; it has no other nutritional advantage.

Raw sugar is sucrose obtained by direct evaporation of sugar cane juice. Unless dirt and other undesirable matter are removed, it is not recommended for human consumption.

Molasses is the residue after the extraction of sugar crystals from the raw sugar plant juice. It is the only sweetener that contains any significant amounts of vitamins (B_6 and other Bs) and minerals (iron, potassium, calcium).

Brown sugar is sucrose (table sugar) combined with molasses syrup.

Honey consists of several sugars, chiefly fructose and glucose, in varying proportions. Because of its high fructose content, it achieves a specific degree of sweetness with somewhat fewer calories than table sugar. Tablespoon for tablespoon, however, honey has more calories. Notwithstanding its reputation, it contains only the barest trace amounts of vitamins and minerals. The color and flavor of honey depend on the flowers on which the bees were feeding.

Lactose, or milk sugar, is found in the milk of mammals and is composed of glucose and galactose. It is made commercially from whey (the watery part of milk), and used in the manufacture of drugs.

Galactose, also known as "brain sugar," is a component of the lactose in milk.

Maltose, or malt sugar, is composed of two glucose molecules. It is formed by fermentation or by chemical means. Maltose is used commercially in foods and drugs.

Corn syrup is produced from cornstarch. The use of sweeteners derived from corn—corn syrup, corn sugar, dextrose—has increased tremendously over the last few decades. Corn syrup consists mostly of fructose and glucose in varying proportions.

Maple syrup is primarily sucrose. When the liquid of the sap is boiled off, maple sugar is produced.

Sorbitol and **mannitol** (technically sugar alcohols) are found in some plants but are also produced commercially from dextrose —to be used, for example, in the manufacture of chewing gum and drug coatings. They are about half as sweet as table sugar. Because sugar alcohols are metabolized differently from other sugars, they are preferred to sugar in food processed for diabetics.

Xylitol (wood sugar), another sugar alcohol, is made from birch wood, but is also found naturally in some fruits and berries. It is approximately as sweet as table sugar and is used like the other sugar alcohols. The safety of xylitol is under investigation.

NON-CALORIC SWEETENERS

With the introduction and increasing popularity of diet soft drinks, artificial sweeteners have come into wider and wider use over the past 35 or 40 years. They are now used by millions of Americans in food, beverages and drugs. Diabetics comprise a small percentage of consumers; the vast majority use the sweeteners for purposes of weight control, although there is in fact no documented evidence that this practice contributes to weight loss in the long run.

Saccharin was discovered in 1879, and proved useful during sugar shortages in World Wars I and II. In recent years several animal studies have cast doubt on the safety of saccharin, specifically when very large amounts are taken. For a time the product was removed from marketed foods and drinks, but it is now available once again, and used quite widely. Sweet'n Low and Sugar Twin are brands that contain saccharin.

Saccharine is 300 times sweeter than an equal weight of sugar. It has no calories.

Cyclamate, discovered about half a century ago, came into wide use in the 1950s and 1960s. In recent years its safety has come under scrutiny, and its use was suspended. It may, however, be permitted again in the near future.

Cyclamate is 30 times sweeter than sugar and has no calories. It is heat stable and dissolves easily in liquid.

Aspartame too has been subjected to a great deal of debate and much testing since it was discovered in 1965. For the last several years it has been approved for use in foods, beverages and drugs. Except in individuals with a rare genetic disease (phenylketonuria, or PKU), it is considered safe when taken in reasonable amounts.

Weight for weight aspartame actually has the same number of calories as sugar, but it is 200 times as sweet, and therefore only tiny amounts are needed. It does not retain this sweetness with prolonged heating, or when in solution for any length of time. The trade name is NutraSweet. It is used in Equal.

Sunette is the trade name of the newest approved artificial sweetener, Acesulfame K. It has no calories, is as sweet as aspartame, and is said to retain its qualities with heating and with prolonged storage. Like the other artificial sweeteners, it will continue to be studied in the coming years.

Several more artificial sweeteners are in the testing stage, among them **Sucralose**, a non-caloric relative of table sugar and 600 times sweeter, and **Alitame,** composed of amino acids and 2,000 times as sweet as sugar.

We may never be entirely certain that any artificial sweetener is totally safe. For the time being, none of them should really be used by children and pregnant women. At the same time, practically speaking, artificial sweeteners are now found in so many foods and beverages that they are almost impossible to avoid.

FIBER

Most dietary fiber—"roughage" or "bulk"—consists of plant material that is indigestible and has no calories. Fiber does, however, affect digestion by drawing water into the stool, softening it and giving it more volume, and by regulating transit time through the intestinal tract. Fiber can also elicit the secretion of intestinal hormones and enzymes, and influence the absorption of nutrients; in that sense it may affect nutrition. Because it has a satiating effect, some dieters find high-fiber foods to be helpful in curbing hunger.

In recent years fiber has been categorized according to solubility in water. Insoluble fiber, mainly cellulose, exerts its action in the lower intestine, providing bulk. Soluble fiber acts on the upper intestine as well. There it affects the absorption of food stuffs and is being promoted as having a cholesterol-lowering effect (perhaps by altering bile acid metabolism).

As an aside, the term "cholesterol lowering" is actually a medical claim, but at present the FDA has only limited jurisdiction over such labeling. As a result, in the last few years 40 percent of new food products introduced to the marketplace made health claims of one sort or another. Fortunately, a new food labeling law is on the horizon. This will require that such claims must be scientifically verified in much the same way that the effectiveness (and safety) of a drug must be proved before it is released to the public.

Insoluble fiber is found in bran, vegetables and fruits. Many fruits and vegetables also contain *soluble* fiber. Among them are the current favorites, oat bran and rice bran. Bran products—eaten in hopes of lowering cholesterol—can be tricky, however. Beware of cereals processed with highly saturated coconut oil, which is likely to *raise* blood cholesterol; and even bran cereals produced with unsaturated fatty acids can derive a third of their calories from fat.*

Fiber supplements have not proved themselves.

Representative items in several food groups are listed on the next page according to relative fiber content.

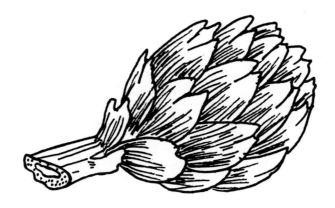

*Example: Kellogg's Cracklin' Oat Bran contains 4g of fat per 110 calorie serving. 4g of fat, at 9 calories per gram, produce 36 calories of fat—which shows fat comprising 33% of the total calories.

	Low Fiber	Medium Fiber	High Fiber
CEREALS	Cream of rice	Oatmeal	Bran
	Cream of wheat	Shredded wheat	(all kinds)
	Farina	Cornflakes	Bran flakes
	Puffed rice	Granola	
	White rice	Brown rice	
		Barley	
BREAD	White	Whole wheat	
	Italian	Pumpernickel	
	French	(If labels	
	Rye	specify whole	
		grain flour)	
VEGETABLES	Strained juice	Lettuce	Artichokes
		Onions	Most beans
		Snap beans	Lentils
		Carrots	Peas
		Tomatoes	Chickpeas
		Peppers	Broccoli
		Spinach	Corn
FRUITS	Strained juice	Bananas	Berries
		Melons	Whole apples
		Applesauce	Whole pears
		Plums	Figs
		Peaches	Dates
		Grapes	Prunes
		Citrus fruit	
		Cherries	
NUTS		Peanuts	Brazil nuts
		Almonds	Coconuts
		Walnuts	

Although there is no specific recommendation regarding amounts, an inadequate intake of fiber in western countries is blamed for various "diseases of civilization," chiefly affecting the bowel. This suspicion is not new. The Greek physician Hippocrates advised that the bran be left in meal (flour) to help bowel function.

A typical Western diet includes about ½ ounce of pure fiber daily, half of it from legumes and vegetables, the other half from cereals and fruits. In less industrialized regions, where plant foods are not highly processed, adults may consume 4 ounces a day or more.

Excessive amounts of fiber can cause rumbling, bloating and diarrhea, and may interfere with the absorption of vitamin B_{12} and some important minerals. The wisest course is to eat a balanced diet that includes fresh fruits, vegetables, and whole grain cereals and bread.

LOW-RESIDUE AND BLAND DIETS

A low-residue diet eliminates foods high in fiber. A *bland* diet is similar to a low-residue diet, but it is also restricted with regard to spices. These diets are designed to soothe the intestinal tract and to lighten the digestive workload. Transit through the bowel is slowed; stools are small and infrequent.

The next page shows a list of foods appropriate for such diets.

Low Residue/Bland Diets

FOODS PERMITTED

- precooked or cooked fine cereals
- noodles and pasta
- white bread
- cream soups
- milk, cream, cottage cheese, yogurt, cream cheese, butter
- margarine, oil
- eggs (not fried)
- potatoes (skinned and not fried), strained or chopped sweet potatoes, squash, carrots
- bananas, cooked fruit without skins
- strained fruit juices
- ground meat, poultry or fish, not fried
- ice cream, fruit gelatin, custard, pudding

FOODS NOT ALLOWED

- whole grain breads and cereals
- meat extract or stock
- processed meats and cheeses
- raw vegetables, cooked cabbage, corn and legumes
- raw fruit, except bananas
- strong spices and flavorings
- nuts
- tea, coffee, carbonated drinks
- any form of alcohol

CEREAL GRAINS

This is a loosely defined group of a number of very important food plants. Technically, most of these crops are actually the seeds of grasses, but one—buckwheat—is a fruit. All are high in carbohydrates. Protein and fat contents vary, and so does the amount of bran. Bran is the chaff or seed covering of cereal plants. It is largely indigestible, but serves as a source of fiber and some B vitamins. Brief descriptions of various plants are given below in alphabetical order. If importance were used as the ranking criterion, wheat, rice and corn would head the list.

Amaranth: a high-protein designer grain, first cultivated by the Aztecs.

Barley: probably the most ancient cultivated cereal grain, with evidence of prehistoric use in China and Egypt. Since Greek and Roman times it has been grown extensively as a source of food and animal feed, and for the production of liquor. Barley corn is a grain of barley. *Pearl barley* has had all outer layers removed from the grain.

Barley and some other grains can be subjected to a special process that produces malt. Malt is used in beer making and also in some foods and drugs.

Buckwheat: a plant that produces kernels known as *groats*. Compared to other crops, groats are rich in amino acids. Roasted groats are sold as *kasha*. Buckwheat is valued because it is very hardy and can be grown in poor soil.

Corn: "the American grain," maize, introduced to Europe by the Spaniards, now an invaluable crop worldwide for food, animal fodder, and for the manufacture of corn oil, corn syrup (a major commercial sweetener), cornstarch, dextrose, and many other food and non-food products.

Hominy consists of hulled kernels. (American Indians did the hulling by soaking corn in a weak lye solution.) Hominy can then be ground to produce *grits*. Bourbon is distilled from a mash that is at least 50 percent corn; corn whiskey contains at least 80 percent corn mash.

Emmer: a hardy European grain closely related to wheat.

Millet: one of the oldest of grains. It is still the food staple of India, and is common in underdeveloped countries and some parts of Europe and Japan.

Oats: a grain grown in temperate and cool climates all over the world. It is used for dry and cooked cereals, and provides important animal fodder that is relatively high in protein, minerals and vitamins. Oat bran, which has become popular of late, supplies water soluble fiber, as opposed to unprocessed wheat bran, which is insoluble.

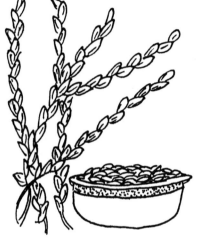

Quinoa: the sacred mother grain of the Incas, still used widely in the Andes. It is high in protein. Quinoa is now increasingly cultivated in the United States where a similar plant, known as lamb's quarters, has long grown wild.

Rice: known for 9,000 years, and cultivated for almost that long. Rice is used as the main dietary staple by more people than any other food. More than 7,000 varieties have been developed. Western countries prefer *long grain* rice. *"Short grain,"* used in Far Eastern countries, is more glutinous or sticky. (Glutinous does not mean that it contains gluten.) Sticky rice is the main component of sushi.

Brown or *unpolished rice* has more vitamins and fiber than polished rice, because the bran remains (after the husk has been removed). *Converted rice* is processed to retain much of the fiber and nutrients. *Instant rice* is precooked,and is the least nutritious. Several foreign grown varieties of rice are now available in the United States in addition to Far Eastern types, among them *Arborio*, a short grain creamy rice from Italy, and *Basmati*, an aromatic white or brown long grain variety from India.

Sake and other alcoholic beverages are made from rice.

Rye: a grain closely related to wheat, most commonly grown in Northern Europe and other cool climates. Because rye does not contain much gluten, it produces a heavy, dense bread. In the United States wheat flour is usually mixed with it to produce a lighter color and texture.

Rye can be fermented to make whiskey.

Sorghum: a plant that resembles corn in appearance. It is used as a forage plant and also for food in the United States, India, China and Africa. Some varieties yield a syrup.

Triticale: a hybrid between wheat and rye that has a high protein content.

Wheat: now the world's largest food crop, used primarily for making flour. Wheat was first grown in the Nile valley, at least 7,000 years ago. About a dozen species and literally thousands of varieties are cultivated, depending on climate,soil, intended use, local disease and pest resistance, and regional preference. *Common wheat,* a species that includes numerous varieties, is the favorite grain for breadmaking, because it contains in its kernel a large quantity of gluten, which helps to make dough rise and gives bread its characteristic texture. Varieties of the *durum* species are used in pasta making, because they allow macaroni products to hold up with cooking. *Semolina* is a purified component of durum. *Graham* flour is whole wheat flour. *Cracked wheat* is wheat that has been dried, and then cracked and ground. *Bulgur wheat* is first cooked, then dried and ground. *Wheat germ,* a part of each wheat kernel, is a substance rich in vitamin E and manganese.

Wheat is used to make beer and whiskey.

Wild rice: a water grass first harvested by American Indians, and now grown commercially.

GLUTEN

Gluten is the insoluble protein ingredient of most grains, including wheat, rye, oats, barley, and buckwheat. It is the material that gives elasticity to dough. In certain disorders of intestinal absorption, gluten must be restricted and the following foods should be avoided:

- noodles and pasta
- most commercial baked goods
- wheat, rye, oat, barley,
    and buckwheat cereals
- processed meats and cheeses
- gravies, sauces and soups made with flour
- breadings and stuffings
- most ice creams
- cocoa mix, malted milk, most syrups
- beer, ale, whiskey

The following foods are permitted on a gluten-restricted diet:

- plain vegetables, fruits and fruit juices
- potatoes and rice
- rice and corn cereals
- baked goods made with potato, rice, corn
  or soy flour
- milk, natural cheese, eggs, butter
- oil, margarine
- meat, fowl, fish, shellfish
- gelatin, sherbet
- honey, jam, jelly, sugar
- coffee, tea, carbonated drinks

A number of companies make gluten-free food products, and they are labeled as such.

OXALIC ACID (OXALATE)

Oxalic acid is a natural component of many plants. Considerable quantities of it are found in the following food items:

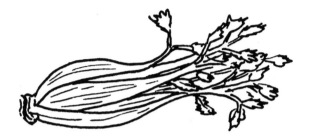

VEGETABLES	Purslane, pokeweed, sorrel, rhubarb, beets, spinach, peppers, parsley, scallions, celery, carrots, artichoke, yams, okra, rhubarb
FRUITS	Plums, red grapes, berries, figs, oranges
MISCELLANEOUS	Instant coffee, cocoa, cola drinks, pecans, peanuts

Even though it is a naturally occurring substance, oxalic acid is potentially harmful; it is present at such low concentrations, however, that it presents no risk of toxicity to healthy individuals when eaten in conventional food portions. When taken in very large quantities, or in certain medical conditions, it can hamper the absorption of important minerals—particularly calcium and magnesium—by combining with them and tying them into unusable oxalate salts.

FASCINATING FACTS
ABOUT CARBOHYDRATES

• "Complex carbohydrates" are foods whose chief component is a form of starch. This includes cereals, breads, pasta, rice, and potatoes. Fruits and green vegetables are primarily complex carbohydrates too, but usually they also contain a significant proportion of fiber. Complex carbohydrates are much in fashion now, just as high-protein foods were in previous decades.

• "Wheat flour" on a label does not mean whole wheat flour. Bread marked 100% whole wheat is made of whole wheat flour, but the term whole wheat bread means very little, unless whole wheat flour is the first listed ingredient. If whole wheat flour is not the main flour used, the dark color of wheat bread usually comes from caramel or molasses, and the bread is nutritionally not superior to white bread.

• Ounce for ounce, prunes have two-thirds the calories of cornflakes and four and a half times as much fiber.

• Consumers concerned about the sugar content of a processed food should add all the different sugars on the ingredient list. Cereals, for example, may contain sugar, brown sugar, dextrose, corn syrup, malt syrup, honey, sucrose etc. Each one may be present in a relatively small amount, and therefore not at the head of the ingredient list, but when all the sugars are added up, they may amount to a whole lot!

• Potatoes often have fewer calories than their various embellishments. A medium baked potato, for instance, provides 95 calories, a tablespoon of butter 108.

CHAPTER III

The Many Faces of Fat

Fats are a major concern today to consumers, nutritionists, basic scientists, and food providers. This chapter is slightly technical in part, for those who want to understand the terms a little more fully.

Fat is the most concentrated source of calories, furnishing more than twice as much energy per unit weight as protein or carbohydrate. Foods with a fat content of 20 to 30 percent, such as certain meats, cold cuts, and cheeses, actually derive more than half their calories from fat. As an example, American cheese contains 30 percent fat, but the fat provides 73 percent of the calories.

Current thinking holds that no more than 30 percent of the day's total calories should be obtained from fat. A 1,700-calorie diet, for example, should contain no more than two ounces of fat; an ounce of pure fat provides 255 calories, so that two ounces would supply 510 calories or 30 percent of the daily caloric intake.

Total fat, moreover, is not the only limiting factor. Fats differ in their health implications. It is recommended that the total fat allowance be divided equally among saturated, monounsaturated, and polyunsaturated fatty acids.

FATS AND FATTY ACIDS

Saturated fats are the fats that have been linked to elevated blood cholesterol and to damaging effects on blood vessels, including those that supply the heart and brain. In a way of explanation, "saturated" means that the fatty acid molecule holds all the hydrogen it can. "Hydrogenation" (often seen on a label) is a process that increases saturation. This is done·to make an oil solid at room temperature, and also to make the product more stable (increase its "shelf life").

Fats are·usually mixtures of several different fatty acids and fatty acid types. As a general rule, the more saturated a fat product is, the more likely will it be solid at room temperature, and also the more stable on heating and prolonged storage. Some fats, such as soybean oil, undergo a degree of hydrogenation on heating. For this reason soybean oil is often sold mixed with corn oil, or it is deliberately partly hydrogenated and then purified; this makes it more suitable for cooking and also retards rancidity.

Saturated fatty acids themselves appear to differ in their effect on blood cholesterol levels. Myristic acid, particularly prominent in butter fat, raises cholesterol more than some others. Stearic acid, found especially in beef and chocolate, may by itself actually lower cholesterol, but unfortunately is present in these foods along with less favorable saturated fatty acids.

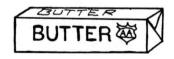

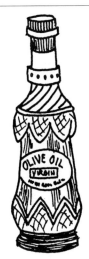

Monounsaturated fatty acids have one double bond, capable of absorbing an additional hydrogen atom. These fatty acids tend to produce a more favorable blood cholesterol profile, namely a lower cholesterol, a higher HDL and a higher HDL/LDL ratio.* Population studies also suggest that monounsaturates help with control of blood sugar in diabetics.

Polyunsaturated fatty acids have two or more double bonds that provide available sites. They, too, play a role in lowering cholesterol and blood sugar. Some of them, moreover, are essential for adequate nutrition; since the human body cannot produce them, they must be included in the diet. (Fats are found in so many varieties of foods however, even many fruits and vegetables, that this rarely presents a problem.)

Nevertheless, despite their good reputation, polyunsaturated fatty acids are not necessarily the unqualified best choice of fat. Since monounsaturated fatty acids have only one available double bond, they invite fewer free radicals upon heating than do the polyunsaturated fatty acids; this is in their favor, because there has been a suggestion that heat-induced free radicals promote tumor growth and impair the immune system. (Antioxidants are advocated to counteract this adverse effect of polyunsaturation.) In any event, monounsaturated oils, such as olive oil, may turn out to be the best choice for cooking.

Shown on the next page in simplified diagram form are prototypes of fatty acid "chains." Actually, the chains can be much longer. Marine polyunsaturates have more than 18 carbon

---

* These terms are defined in the lipoprotein section.

atoms; 25 to 30 percent of the chains have as many as 20 or 22 carbons, and as many as 6 double bonds, indicating a high degree of unsaturation. Mammalian and most vegetable fats have fewer long chains and fewer double bonds, and the double bonds occur at different sites.

Saturated fatty acids have no double carbon-carbon bonds; that is, the carbon atoms (C) are connected to each other with single bonds (–).

$$
\cdots-\overset{\overset{\textstyle H}{|}}{\underset{\underset{\textstyle H}{|}}{C}}-\overset{\overset{\textstyle H}{|}}{\underset{\underset{\textstyle H}{|}}{C}}-\overset{\overset{\textstyle H}{|}}{\underset{\underset{\textstyle H}{|}}{C}}-\overset{\overset{\textstyle H}{|}}{C}-\cdots
$$

Monounsaturated fatty acids have one double bond (=) where hydrogen atoms (H) could otherwise be attached.

$$
\cdots-\overset{\overset{\textstyle H}{|}}{\underset{\underset{\textstyle H}{|}}{C}}-\overset{\overset{\textstyle H}{|}}{\underset{\underset{\textstyle H}{|}}{C}}-\overset{\overset{\textstyle H}{|}}{C}=\overset{\overset{\textstyle H}{|}}{C}-\overset{\overset{\textstyle H}{|}}{\underset{\underset{\textstyle H}{|}}{C}}-\overset{\overset{\textstyle H}{|}}{\underset{\underset{\textstyle H}{|}}{C}}-\cdots
$$

Polyunsaturated fatty acids have two or more double bonds.

$$
\cdots-\overset{\overset{\textstyle H}{|}}{\underset{\underset{\textstyle H}{|}}{C}}-\overset{\overset{\textstyle H}{|}}{C}=\overset{\overset{\textstyle H}{|}}{C}-\overset{\overset{\textstyle H}{|}}{\underset{\underset{\textstyle H}{|}}{C}}-\overset{\overset{\textstyle H}{|}}{C}=\overset{\overset{\textstyle H}{|}}{C}-\overset{\overset{\textstyle H}{|}}{\underset{\underset{\textstyle H}{|}}{C}}-\cdots
$$

Fatty acids can also be described with simple monograms which indicate the length of the carbon chain, the number of double bonds, and the location of the first of these double bonds from the end of the chain. For example, C18:2n-6 means an 18-carbon chain with 2 double bonds, the first of them at the 6th carbon (the n-6 or omega-6 position). Fish oils—much in the news—are n-3 fatty acids.

THE DIFFERENT OILS AND FATS

The table on the following page delineates the fatty acid content of the various familiar fats and oils and indicates which ones contain cholesterol.

	SFA	MONO	PUFA	
		(as percent of total fat)		
OILS				
Canola oil	6	62	32	Lowest in SFA
Coconut oil	84	11	1	Highest in SFA
Cod-liver oil	8	49	37	X
Corn oil	13	25	62	
Cottonseed oil	27	19	54	
Olive oil	13	76	9	Highest in MONO
Palm kernel oil	79	16	2	Very high in SFA
Palm oil	48	40	9	
Peanut oil	17	50	32	
Safflower oil	10	14	75	Highest in PUFA
Sesame oil	14	42	43	
Soybean oil	16	23	61	
Sunflower oil	12	19	68	
Walnut oil	9	18	73	
Wheat germ oil	29	18	53	
FATS				
Beef fat	50	46	4	X
Butter	60	36	4	X
Chicken fat	30	49	21	X
Lard (pork fat)	39	50	11	X
Margarine (average)	19	53	27	
Vegetable shortening	29	44	27	

SFA = saturated fatty acids
MONO = monounsaturated fatty acids
PUFA = polyunsaturated fatty acids
X = contains cholesterol

CHOLESTEROL AND SATURATED FAT

Cholesterol is not a fat in the usual sense, but a waxy substance that is a component of all animal tissue and all animal fats. In our bodies it plays a vital role in the stability of cells and the structure of cell membranes. It is also a necessary building block for a number of hormones. Ordinarily about a third of our cholesterol comes from food, the rest is made by our own cells, chiefly in the liver. After infancy no cholesterol needs to be included in the diet, because the body produces all it needs.

We hear a great deal about cholesterol nowadays, because studies have shown that there is an association between high levels of cholesterol in the blood and the probability of a heart attack and other medical problems. It is important, however, not to confuse cholesterol in the blood with the cholesterol that we eat. Cholesterol in food does have an impact on blood cholesterol, but it is only one of many factors, not all of which we can entirely control. Although we cannot change heredity, which is a powerful determinant, even unfavorable genetics can be modified by a sensible lifestyle and diet: we certainly can determine the type of food we eat.

Current thinking holds that we should limit our cholesterol intake to about 300 mg a day; and, just as important, no more than 10 percent of our calories should come from saturated fatty acids. Eating saturated fats is more apt to raise the blood cholesterol than will eating cholesterol itself. (A definition of saturated fat is found in the section on fats and fatty acids.)

Unlike cholesterol, saturated fats may be of animal or vegetable origin. Pastries and cookies, made with saturated vegetable fats (and cholesterol-free), will raise the blood cholesterol in susceptible individuals.

In animal products, fat is often visible to the naked eye. This is fat, not cholesterol.

There is great variation in the saturated fat content of meat, depending on the amount of visible fat and the marbling of the meat. (The choicest, most tender cuts often contain the most marbling, and therefore the most fat.)

Cholesterol is invisible and is found even in lean muscle tissue; that pertains not only to meat and poultry, but also to fish and shellfish. The differences between beef and veal, or between meat, poultry, and seafood, lie chiefly in their saturated fat content, rather than in the amount of cholesterol they contain.

Saturated Fat and Cholesterol Content in Comparable Portions of Meat, Poultry and Seafood

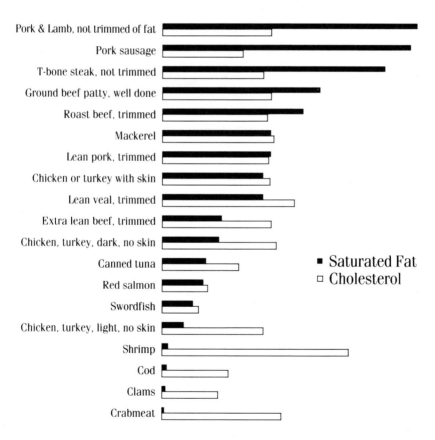

It is hard to say what a normal blood cholesterol is. For one thing, we must not confuse "normal" with "average," because the average in Western society is now considered too high; and for another, what is usually measured is total cholesterol, which is not necessarily the most significant assessment. (This is discussed further under "Lipoproteins" and under "Cardiovascular Risk"). Broadly speaking, and without regard to age or sex or ever-changing opinions and guidelines, it is best to aim for a total blood cholesterol below 200 mg* percent.

Listed below and on the following pages are average portions of some common food items, their caloric value (CAL), the number of calories provided by saturated fat (SAT FAT CAL), and the cholesterol content (CHOL) measured in milligrams. (Cholesterol cannot be said to have calories.) All values are approximate. No allowances are made for fat that may be added in cooking or serving.

To reiterate current guidelines: limiting saturated fat intake is at least as important as limiting cholesterol. Saturated fat calories should not exceed one-tenth of total calories, and therefore should range from 100 to 300 calories daily, depending on one's total caloric requirement.

One ounce of any kind of fat supplies about 250 calories.

	CAL	SAT FAT CAL	CHOL (mg)
MEAT: 3.5 oz (100 gms) cooked weight			
Beef, extra lean, trimmed of fat	190	25	90
Ground beef patty	280	65	90
Roast beef, trimmed of visible fat	242	58	87
T-bone steak, "choice," not trimmed	330	92	84
Beef liver	161	17	420

---

*200 mg percent is the standard way of saying that a substance comprises two-tenths of a percent of the total (two parts in a thousand).

(Continued)	CAL	SAT FAT CAL	CHOL (mg)
Veal rump roast, lean only	156	42	118
Veal blade (breast meat), not trimmed	250	90	90
Lamb leg roast, lean only	191	27	99
Lamb rib chop meat, not trimmed	344	120	90
Pork tenderloin, lean only	166	15	91
Pork loin, lean only	240	45	89
Pork loin chop meat, not trimmed	390	103	90
Ham, cured, boneless	215	32	92
Pork sausage	389	100	68
Chicken or turkey, light, no skin	170	10	84
Chicken or turkey, dark, no skin	194	24	95
Chicken or turkey with skin (avg)	244	42	90
Chicken liver	205	16	550
Brains	100	19	1,960

PROCESSED MEAT: 2 oz (58 gms)

	CAL	SAT FAT CAL	CHOL (mg)
Bologna (2 or 3 slices)	178	60	32
Boiled ham, very lean, 2 slices	78	10	26
Turkey bologna	140	26	57
Turkey ham	73	9	34
Liverwurst	190	55	88
Salami, dry hard (5 or 6 slices)	400	105	48
Frankfurter, beef and/or pork	180	54	34
Frankfurter, chicken or turkey	134	29	52

FISH AND SHELLFISH: 3.5 oz (100 gms)

	CAL	SAT FAT CAL	CHOL (mg)
Caviar	260	90	300
Clams (meat)	120	2	47
Cod	105	2	55
Crabmeat	102	2	100
Haddock	80	2	60
Halibut	100	4	50

(Continued)	CAL	SAT FAT CAL	CHOL (mg)
Lobster meat	92	1	85
Mackerel	198	45	93
Oysters (meat)	66	0	50
Salmon, red	175	17	36
Shrimp	100	3	155
Swordfish	155	13	30
Tuna, canned in oil	198	18	65
Pink salmon, canned	140	14	35

DAIRY PRODUCTS, EGGS AND SUBSTITUTES

	CAL	SAT FAT CAL	CHOL (mg)
Whole milk, 3½ % butterfat, 8 oz.	150	46	33
Skim milk, 8 oz	86	3	5
Heavy cream, 1 oz	100	60	40
Evaporated milk, 1 oz	42	13	10
Non-dairy creamer, soybean oil, 1 oz	40	5	0
Non-dairy creamer, coconut/palm oil, 1 oz	40	25	0
Butter, 1 tbs	108	68	32
Margarine, corn oil, stick, 1 tbs	108	22	0
Ice cream, 16% fat, ½ cup	175	66	44
Ice cream, 10% fat, ½ cup	135	40	30
Yogurt, whole milk, 8 oz	148	43	29
Yogurt, low fat, 8 oz	140	21	14
Cottage cheese, ½ cup	117	29	24
Cottage cheese, 1% butterfat, ½ cup	82	6	12
Cheese, part skim, 2 oz	144	52	32
Cheddar, blue, cream cheese, 2 oz	230	109	62
American, Swiss, feta, Parmesan, 2 oz	180	72	50
American non-fat (Kraft Free)	90	0	10
Eggs, 2 large	158	31	426
Eggbeaters, equivalent of 2 eggs	50	0	0
Tofutti Egg Watchers, equivalent of 2 eggs	100	5	0

(Continued)	CAL	SAT FAT CAL	CHOL (mg)
Scramblers, equivalent of 2 eggs	120	18	0
Egg yolks, 2 large	125	31	426
Egg whites, 2 large	33	0	0

FATS, OILS, DRESSINGS, SPREADS: 1 tbs

	CAL	SAT FAT CAL	CHOL (mg)
Lard	116	45	15
Beef tallow	116	58	14
Codliver oil	120	10	81
Coconut oil	120	106	0
Other oils—(see Different Oils. . .)	120		
Vegetable shortening	106	29	0
Non-stick spray (1½ seconds)	8	2	0
Oil/vinegar dressing	70	9	0
Hollandaise and similar sauces	45	24	12
Gravy, canned	12	2	1
Mayonnaise	100	18	5
Peanut butter	94	14	0
Jam or jelly	55	0	0

VEGETABLES, FRUITS, NUTS

(Vegetable products do not contain cholesterol. Most fruits and vegetables also contain no saturated fat; some that do are listed below.)

	CAL	SAT FAT CAL	CHOL (mg)
Avocado, ½ large	230	32	0
Banana, medium	105	2	0
Chickpeas, 4 oz, canned	205	4	0
Coconut meat, 1 oz	102	78	0
Olives, 2 oz (10–12 large)	110	9	0
Peanuts, 1 oz	170	28	0
Pumpkin seeds, 1 oz	157	21	0
Tofu	85	7	0
Wheat germ, 1 oz	108	5	0

(Continued)	CAL	SAT FAT CAL	CHOL (mg)

BAKED GOODS, CEREALS, PASTA, SWEETS

(Baked goods vary widely, depending on inclusion of eggs and milk, as well as type and quantity of fat. Estimates are given.)

	CAL	SAT FAT CAL	CHOL (mg)
Bagel	200	3	0
Bread, white or whole wheat, 1 slice	70	3	1
Biscuit, 1 oz, from mix	93	5	2
Biscuit, 1 oz, lard or solid shortening	103	6	15
Corn muffin	145	14	23
Croissant, large	235	32	13
English muffin	140	3	0
Hamburger or hot dog bun	115	5	1
Popover	112	15	71
Ritz crackers, 5 pieces	90	12	3
Saltines, 5 pieces	65	4	0
Corn flakes, 1 cup (0.8 oz)	94	0	0
Granola, 1 cup	505	52	0
Oatmeal, ¾ cup (1 oz dry)	108	3	0
Spaghetti, cooked, 1 cup	190	2	0
Egg noodles, cooked, 1 cup	160	6	50
Angel food cake, slice	125	0	0
Chocolate chip cookie	46	12	9
Chocolate cake with icing, 3 oz	310	65	36
Doughnut, plain	210	24	20
Fruit cake, 1½ oz	167	22	27
Lemon meringue pie, ⅙ of 9" pie	355	39	143
Sponge cake, 3 oz	235	14	201
Milk chocolate, 1 oz	142	54	6

LIPOPROTEINS

Since fats will not dissolve in blood, which is a watery substance, they must be transported through the bloodstream, piggyback, by other compounds. These compounds are the lipoproteins, complex combinations of proteins and fats. Among them are the high density lipoproteins (HDL), low density lipoproteins (LDL), and very low density lipoproteins (VLDL). In accordance with their different structures, they carry different proportions of cholesterol and triglycerides, and they have different functions. Triglycerides are carried mainly by VLDL and make up the greatest part of that molecule. About two-thirds of all cholesterol is transported by LDL.

Stated in simplified terms, LDL and VLDL are bad, because they encourage deposition of fatty material in the walls of blood vessels and therefore contribute to the risk of heart disease. HDL is good because it removes cholesterol from tissues, mostly to be disposed of by the liver. (Unfortunately HDLs do not occur as such in foods; they must be manufactured by the body, rather than eaten.) Exercise, female hormones, and a diet low in saturated fat and cholesterol all contribute to raising HDL. Incidentally, the term density (as in high or low density) is related to the laboratory method that is used in lipoprotein testing.

Lipoprotein testing has assumed an important role in recent years. Many physicians and scientist now think that, for the purpose of assessing cardiovascular risk, measuring total cholesterol (TC) is not nearly as revealing as measuring lipoprotein fractions. A low or normal TC composed mainly of LDL-cholesterol and VLDL-cholesterol may be more ominous than a TC that is slightly elevated but has a high HDL-cholesterol portion. In other words, it is the ratios as well as the absolute numbers that are significant in risk assessment. Of all the tests related to cholesterol, the percentage of HDL may be the best predictive indicator.

Desirable values are different for men and women and for different ages. Nevertheless, the values shown below may be useful, if they are taken as approximations rather than firm guidelines. They apply to adults only.

Lab Test	Desirable Value
TC	less than 200 mg %*
LDL	less than 130 mg %
HDL	more than 45 mg %
TC/HDL	less than 3.5
%HDL (100 x HDL/TC)	more than 28
Triglycerides	less than 160 mg %

TRIGLYCERIDES

Triglycerides are fatty substances normally present in the blood. They are carried as part of the lipoprotein molecule, chiefly on VLDL (see Lipoproteins). There is uncertainty about the significance of slightly elevated triglycerides; it may or may not represent a risk factor for heart disease in otherwise healthy women; in men there is even less of a correlation. Very high triglycerides often indicate an inborn abnormality or they reflect an underlying illness; in any event, marked elevation does indeed pose a threat, and medical intervention is advisable.

Best values are below 160 mg percent, with blood drawn in the fasting state.

---

* A mg % is a thousandth of a percent, or one part in a hundred thousand.

FISH AND FISH OIL

Although Eskimos eat a diet high in animal fat and cholesterol and low in vegetables and vegetable fats, they have a lower rate of heart disease than other North Americans whose average diet consists of less fat and more carbohydrate. Current thinking attributes this to the *type* of fat found in fish, seal, and whale meat. Even though this fat is obviously of animal origin, and therefore contains cholesterol, it is indirectly derived from cold-water plants, and it remains liquid at very low temperatures. Not surprisingly, it is the fish from the coldest waters (particularly the North Atlantic) that is richest in these fats.

The substances most specifically involved are two polyunsaturated so-called omega-3 fatty acids, EPA and DHA (full names: eicosopentaenoic acid and docosahexaenoic acid). "Omega-3" refers to the location of the carbon-carbon double bond (=) closest to the end of the fatty acid chain. (See "Fats and Fatty Acids") The best source of omega-3 fatty acids are the oilier fish, such as mackerel, herring, sardines, salmon, sturgeon, and carp.

The benefits of omega-3 fatty acids appear to be related to several effects: they reduce the stickiness of blood (by reducing blood platelet activity in various ways), they lower cholesterol and triglycerides in the blood, and they improve the ratio between "good" cholesterol (HDL) and "bad" cholesterol (LDL). The first of these effects is probably the most important; however, it is also the one that should mitigate against excessive intake of these fatty acids, since adequate platelet activity is required to prevent abnormal bleeding.

It must be remembered that, like other animal products, seafood contains cholesterol. This is true also of fish oils; a tablespoon of cod liver oil contains more than twice as much cholesterol as butter. Fish oil supplements have not yet been fully accepted as a good substitute for real fish. They should be used only under medical supervision.

Incidentally, some vegetables also contain omega-3 fatty-acids, but these differ from marine fatty acids in molecule size. Their value in the diet has not been determined. The richest plant source is purslane, a vegetable in most common use in the Eastern Mediterranean. Most vegetable oils are primarily omega-6 fatty acids, but recent work suggests that some of them, especially soybean oil, can be partly converted by the body to the omega-3 variety.

$$H-\underset{\underset{H}{|}}{\overset{\overset{H}{|}}{C}}-\underset{\underset{H}{|}}{\overset{\overset{H}{|}}{C}}-\overset{\overset{H}{|}}{C}=\overset{\overset{H}{|}}{C}-\underset{\underset{H}{|}}{\overset{\overset{H}{|}}{C}}-\ldots\ldots\ldots \qquad H-\underset{\underset{H}{|}}{\overset{\overset{H}{|}}{C}}-\underset{\underset{H}{|}}{\overset{\overset{H}{|}}{C}}-\underset{\underset{H}{|}}{\overset{\overset{H}{|}}{C}}-\underset{\underset{H}{|}}{\overset{\overset{H}{|}}{C}}-\overset{\overset{H}{|}}{C}=\overset{\overset{H}{|}}{C}-\underset{\underset{H}{|}}{\overset{\overset{H}{|}}{C}}-\ldots\ldots$$

omega-3 position   **omega-6 position**

Consumers have at times questioned the safety of fish. It is true that fish and shellfish are not subjected to the same inspection routines by the USDA as are meat and poultry. However, a voluntary collaboration of the Food Marketing Institute and the National Marine Fisheries Service does its own evaluation for freshness and cleanliness. (Their seal should be displayed at reliable seafood counters.)

Toxic chemicals from polluted waters and fish toxins are separate problems. Fish toxins particularly are often undetectable by chemical tests; these are substances ingested by the fish which are poisonous to man but not to the fish itself. In general, deep sea fish is safest. When buying fish that comes from ocean reefs or from possibly polluted waters, it is best to buy young, small lean fish; these are less likely to have stored large quantities of chemicals or toxin in their muscle mass. All these warnings notwithstanding, fish and shellfish, when bought at a reliable store, should be considered safe and healthy foods.

At present the average American outside Alaska consumes ten times as much meat as fish.

HIGH-FAT FOODS

Listed below are a few selected foods that derive a large part of their calories from fat.

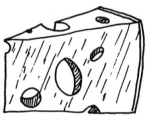

	Approximate Percentage of Calories from Fat
Butter	100
Margarine	100
Oil	100
Vegetable shortening	100
Mayonnaise	99
Heavy cream	97
Macadamia nuts	94
Cream cheese	90
Light cream	90
Salad dressing (avg)	90
Greek olives	89
Sour cream	86
Beef frankfurter	82
Baking chocolate	77
Half & half	77
Peanuts and peanut butter	76
Sunflower seeds	76
American cheese	76
Cheddar cheese	74

(Continued)	Approximate Percentage of Calories from Fat
Avocado	72
Chicken frankfurter	68
Liquid non-dairy creamer	68
T-bone steak, trimmed	65
Egg	64
Pork loin	64
Vanilla ice cream (16% fat)	61
Partially defatted peanuts	60
Cream of mushroom soup (made with milk)	60
Raised doughnut	58
Piecrust	57
Potato chips	57
Croissant	55
Milk chocolate	54
Tofu (soybean curd)	53
Ritz cracker	50
Granola	50

FAST FOODS AND SNACK FOODS

The following list gives the approximate caloric value and the number of calories provided by fat in some common fast foods and snack foods.

	Total Calories	Calories from Fat	Percentage Calories from Fat
ARBY'S			
Roast beef sandwich	350	135	39
Super roast beef sandwich	620	252	41

(Continued)	Total Calories	Calories from Fat	Percentage Calories from Fat
BURGER KING			
Hamburger	290	117	40
Whopper	630	324	51
Whopper with cheese	740	405	55
French fries	210	99	47
Onion rings	270	144	53
DAIRY QUEEN			
Cheese dog	330	171	52
Banana split	540	135	25
Large cone	340	90	26
Medium shake	600	180	30
KENTUCKY FRIED CHICKEN			
Chicken filet sandwich	436	203	47
3-piece dinner, extra crispy (chicken, potato, slaw, roll)	1,070	558	52
McDONALD'S			
Quarter-pounder	420	195	46
Quarter-pounder with cheese	524	276	53
Big Mac	563	297	53
Chicken McNuggets, 6 pieces	314	170	54
Egg McMuffin	327	133	41
PIZZA HUT			
½ of 13″ pizza, thin crust	850	234	28
TACO BELL			
Beef burrito	466	189	41
Taco	162	77	48
WENDY'S			
Hamburger	440	216	49
Double cheeseburger	800	432	54
Chili	230	72	31

(Continued)	Total Calories	Calories from Fat	Percentage Calories from Fat
SARA LEE croissant, 1.5 oz	170	81	58
LAY'S potato chips, 1 oz	149	86	57
FRITOS corn chips, 1 oz	155	87	56
PEPPERIDGE FARM			
Chocolate chip cookie,			
1 piece	160	66	41
Granola cookie, 1 piece	159	69	41
Goldfish, 12 pieces	30	18	60
FROZEN DESSERTS:			
HÄAGEN-DAZS ice cream,			
4 oz	270	153	57
TOFUTTI, 4 oz	230	126	55
ELAN frozen yogurt, 4 oz	125	27	22
TUSCAN yogurt pop, 2.5 oz	130	63	48
TOFULITE choc. frozen			
bar, 3.2 oz	240	135	56
JELL-O vanilla pudding pop	70	18	26
WEIGHT WATCHERS			
sandwich bar	150	27	18
VITARI frozen dessert, 4 oz	80	0	0
Milk chocolate, 2.5 oz (avg)	379	192	51
Carob bar, 2.5 oz	350	171	49
Popcorn, plain, 1 cup	54	6	11
Roasted peanuts, 1 oz	170	126	74
Roasted peanuts, defatted,			
1 oz	154	90	58

LECITHIN

There are several lecithins. They are sticky waxy substances found in cells throughout the body. Lecithin is particularly important in the structure of nerve tissue and its coverings.

Lecithins mix readily with water, and can change the physical texture of fat, homogenizing it into a more liquid state. This property is utilized not only in the body, but also commercially, in the manufacture of ice cream, chocolate, baked goods, and many other foods.

When produced as a health food supplement, lecithin is usually an extract of soybeans. It may also be derived from other fat sources, such as egg yolks and milk. As a nutritional supplement lecithin has been advocated in the treatment of memory loss, as well as for several specific neurologic and psychiatric illnesses. It has also been recommended for the prevention of hardening of the arteries and high blood pressure, and particularly for lowering blood cholesterol. None of these claims has ever been substantiated in controlled studies. The one thing lecithin supplements do is to add calories to the diet.

Estimated Daily Requirement: not known
Estimated average daily intake: 10 grams
Richest sources: Soybeans
Legumes
Egg yolks
Brains

There are no known lecithin-deficiency symptoms in humans.

Toxic effects of lecithin have not been proved, but there have been reports of depression, headache, gastrointestinal symptoms, and rash when lecithin supplements exceeded 30 grams daily.

CHOLINE

Choline is an essential nutrient for some animals, but humans not only get considerable amounts in the diet—in free form and as an integral component of lecithin—but they can also synthesize it. There should be no concern about any specific intake, except perhaps during rapid growth.

Choline is an ingredient of several important bodily substances, concerned particularly with nerve transmission and with the maintenance of cell membranes.

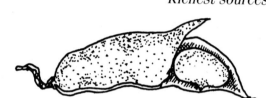

Richest sources: *Egg yolk*
Soybeans
Grains and legumes
Peanuts
Liver

There is no established minimum requirement and there are no recognized deficiency diseases or toxicity. Choline is being added to infant formulas to bring them up to the standard of human milk. Supplements are also being tried to improve memory in the elderly and to treat alcoholic liver disease.

Average daily intake: 500 to 900 mg

Large supplemental doses of choline can cause salivation, nausea and sweating and give the body a fishy odor.

Choline is sometimes classified as a vitamin, but this is not justified.

ARTIFICIAL FAT

We have entered the era of low-calorie and non-caloric fat substitutes. Some day they may become as commonplace as the non-caloric sweeteners that serve as sugar substitutes.

Tests on safety and palatability are being conducted by several companies and scientific groups. The following two products seem to be promising candidates:

Simplesse (NutraSweet/Monsanto), a recently approved product, is made from milk and egg white. It has 15 percent of the calories of regular fat. Simplesse is not intended for cooking or frying, but rather for incorporation into high-fat foods such as cheese.

Olestra (Procter & Gamble), not yet approved, is made from table sugar (sucrose) and several oils, combined into a molecule that cannot be absorbed by the gastrointestinal tract. It will probably be used initially as a partial component of conventional fats used for cooking and frying.

Compounds of similar composition are also being tested as moisture barriers, coating some foods to keep moisture out (crackers, etc.), and some to keep moisture in (produce).

FASCINATING FACTS ABOUT FAT

- Ounce for ounce, cheddar cheese contains more cholesterol than steak, and three times as much saturated fat.

- Coconut oil contains 50% more saturated fat than butter and more than twice as much as lard.

- Cod-liver oil contains two and a half times as much cholesterol as butter.

- Unsaturated fat contains just as many calories as saturated fat.

- Margarine has just as many calories as butter.

- Liquid non-dairy creamer has just as many calories as half-and-half, and, if made with coconut oil, contains more saturated fat.

- "Light" vegetable oil contains as many calories as the regular variety. The "light" label advertises taste.

- Labels that read "pure vegetable oil—no cholesterol" may deceive the unwary into believing that the product is nutritionally superior, but that isn't necessarily so! Vegetable products *never* contain cholesterol, but they may contain a lot of saturated fat if tropical oils are among the ingredients.

- Equally confusing in its implication is "cholesterol-free" mayonnaise, because mayonnaise contains very little cholesterol to begin with! The caloric reduction in "light" mayonnaise is more meaningful. For the sake of comparison, three types of mayonnaise are listed below. Values apply to one tablespoon.

	CALORIES	% FAT CALS	CHOLESTEROL
Regular mayonnaise	100	99	5 mg
Cholesterol-free	90	99	–0–
Reduced-calorie, "light"	50	91	9 mg

• Half the fat in chicken and turkey is in the skin or right beneath it. (This is not true for cholesterol.)

• There is no evidence that eating at bedtime leads to fat deposition, or that exercise after eating prevents it. When it comes to weight changes, the determining factors in healthy individuals are caloric intake and caloric expenditure, regardless of time of day.

CHAPTER IV

Vitamins, Some Real, Some Fanciful

V itamins are complex organic compounds that must be provided in the diet to facilitate a variety of metabolic processes. The human body cannot produce these essential substances, or it produces inadequate amounts, even though only very small quantities are involved.

Vitamins do not contribute any calories.

A "balanced diet" is likely to supply sufficient amounts of vitamins, but many diets are imperfect, and in such cases vitamin supplements may be helpful. However, unless there are specific indications to the contrary, no single ingredient of such a supplement should much exceed its Recommended Daily Dietary Allowance (RDA).

Vitamins are classified as "fat soluble" or "water soluble." This is noteworthy only because fat soluble vitamins require some fat in the diet to be absorbed. Vitamins A, D, E, and K fall into this group. The B vitamins and vitamin C, on the other hand, are water soluble and therefore easily absorbed. By the same token, however, they are also readily excreted and a daily intake is advisable. The fat soluble vitamins are stored in the body to some degree.

Cooking, processing and prolonged storage can cause a loss of some C and B vitamins, but are not as likely to affect the fat soluable ones.

There are eight essential B vitamins: thiamin (B_1), riboflavin (B_2), niacin (B_3), pyridoxine (B_6), vitamin B_{12}, folate, biotin, and pantothenic acid. Several other substances lay claim to being B vitamins, among them choline, PABA, inositol, and pangamic acid, but these substances do not fulfill the criteria of vitamins.

VITAMIN A (RETINOL and BETA-CAROTENE)

Vitamin A is fat soluble, which allows for some degree of storage (chiefly in the liver). This vitamin is essential in many processes. It promotes normal growth and bone formation, maintains good vision, produces healthy skin and mucous membranes, helps avert infection, and, as an antioxidant, plays an important protective role against environmental toxins and cancer-causing agents.

The vitamin A in our diet is derived from two different food groups. Animal products give us retinol, a ready-made vitamin A. Plants supply beta-carotene, which is then converted to vitamin A in the body. In a balanced diet these sources are about equally represented.

Vitamin A nomenclature can be confusing. One microgram of vitamin A is now expressed as one RE (retinol equivalent). It has the same potency as 6 mcg of beta-carotene.

Recommended Dietary Allowance
                    Men: 1,000 RE
                Women: 800 RE

International units (IU) are rarely used anymore. The RDA expressed in IUs is 5,000 for men and 4,000 for women.

Deficiency occurs when there is general malnutrition, or with impaired fat absorption, or when the diet is specifically restricted with regard to vitamin A, such as may be seen in societies where rice is the main food source. In malnourished children vitamin A deficiency most often results from a lack of milk, eggs, and other protein foods, rather than a low beta-carotene intake.

Deficiency leads to night blindness, dry eyes, thickened skin and recurrent infections. In children there is impaired growth, and the eye effects may ultimately lead to blindness.

Richest sources: Fish liver oils
                Liver
                Yellow vegetables
                    (carrots, yams,
                        pumpkins)
                Dark green vegetables
                Fortified dairy products
                Egg yolks
                Fleshy fruits
                    (melons, peaches, apricots).

Toxicity can be a serious problem. Except in specific and supervised situations, vitamin A supplements should not exceed the daily requirement. Excessive amounts over a period of time can result in dry peeling skin, hair loss, blurred vision, bone and joint pain, headache, irritability, abdominal pain, and liver damage. Taken during pregnancy, large doses can lead to abnormalities in the offspring. In young children toxic amounts of vitamin A can actually *retard* growth and mental development. Excess *must* be avoided.

By contrast, beta-carotene in the form of yellow vegetables can be eaten in large amounts as part of the diet, because the conversion to vitamin A is limited by need; the only adverse effect will be yellowing of the skin until the big doses are discontinued.

Vitamin A derivatives are useful in the treatment of several skin conditions, but should never be used without medical supervision.

VITAMIN D (CHOLECALCIFEROL, CALCIFEROL)

Vitamin D is one of the fat-soluble vitamins; because it is fat-soluble, fat is required for its absorption and the vitamin is stored to some degree (chiefly in the liver). Vitamin D regulates growth and bone repair and helps to control the proper hardness of bone and teeth. It also participates in important reactions in the liver and kidneys. All these activities are closely tied to the vitamin's role in the absorption and regulation of calcium and phosphorus (phosphate).

Recommended Dietary Allowances of cholecalciferol
Ages 19–24: 10 mcg
Ages 25 plus: 5 mcg

10 mcg cholecalciferol is equivalent to 400 I.U. of vitamin D (which is the older nomenclature).

In children, deficiency causes irritability, muscle spasms, and the retarded and defective growth pattern known as rickets. Although sunlight is the best generator of vitamin D, rickets is not rare in tropical and subtropical climates. There can be several reasons for this: one, infants in tropical areas are often swaddled and kept indoors; two, the sun is avoided for the sake of appearance; and three, dark skin does not absorb sunlight as well as light skin. In northern countries where sunlight is scarcer, rickets occurs in regions where milk is not fortified with vitamin D.

Vitamin D deficiency in adults causes softening of bones and teeth, poor muscle tone, and impaired kidney function.

Richest sources: Sunlight effect on the skin
Fortified dairy products
and margarine
Fish liver oil
Fish
Egg yolk

Excessive doses of vitamin D, usually in the form of supplements, can have serious consequences, particularly in children. There may be permanent damage to the heart and kidneys, in children and adults, at only five times the recommended dose. Lesser symptoms include weakness, thirst, loss of appetite, vomiting, and headache.

VITAMIN E

Vitamin E comprises a group of oily substances, of which alpha-tocopherol is the most active and the most available in nature. Because vitamin E is fat soluble, it is stored in the body to some degree.

It has long been known that this vitamin is needed by many animal species, and that serious deficiency symptoms occur when it is withheld. In human beings, deficiency has been seen only with illnesses that interfere with normal fat absorption, and in premature infants.

Deficiencies aside, vitamin E is primarily an antioxidant, trapping free radicals and protecting cells and cell membranes. It does this in collaboration with selenium, vitamin C and vitamin A. Numerous other claims have been made for vitamin E by proponents who believe that large amounts are valuable, even though no deficiency can be demonstrated. Vitamin E is being advocated to enhance fertility (tocopherol actually means oil of fertility), to improve sexual potency, to slow down the aging process, to prevent cancer, heart attacks and lung clots, and to treat ulcers, breast cysts, skin diseases and poor circulation. None of these claims has been proved in a controlled setting, but many serious studies are in progress, and it is possible that the RDA will be increased someday.

Recommended Dietary Allowances
Men: 10 α-TE
Women: 8 α-TE

Perplexing as all the health claims are, the nomenclature, as found on food products and vitamin supplements, is even more confusing. The unit used here, α-TE, stands for alpha-Tocopherol Equivalent. One α-TE is equal to the activity of 1 mg d-α-tocopherol, also known as RRR-α-tocopherol. This is the naturally occurring form of the compound. The synthetic form is dl-α-tocopherol; it is 26 percent less active (d and l are mirror forms of a molecule, d standing for right and l for left.) One mg of dl-α-tocopherols is equivalent to 1 IU, which is yet another designation. If a label uses IUs, the RDA should be 14 for men and 11 for women.

> *Richest sources: Wheat germ oil*
> *Other vegetable oils*
> *Nuts and seeds*
> *Green vegetables*
> *Egg yolk*
> *Butter*

A diet very high in polyunsaturated fatty acids may require larger than average doses of vitamin E, even though such fats are themselves good sources of the vitamin.

Large doses are well tolerated. People who take twenty or thirty times the recommended dose seem to have no problems. Hair loss, fatigue, muscle weakness, and diarrhea have been reported with even greater amounts.

VITAMIN K

Vitamin K is a fat-soluble vitamin, necessary for the normal clotting of blood. Human requirements are very small and are generally met by the average diet. A form of vitamin K is also produced by the intestine, but it is uncertain how much of that is utilized.

Recommended Dietary Allowances
Men aged 19–24: 70 mcg
Men aged 25 plus: 80 mcg
Women aged 19–24: 60 mcg
Women aged 25 plus: 65 mcg

Excessive bleeding ensues when there is a significant deficiency of vitamin K. Such a deficiency is most likely to occur in the newborn (whose diet is inadequate and whose intestine is not yet geared up to produce the vitamin), and in individuals with disfunction of the liver or intestine.

Richest sources: Green vegetables
Green tea
Soybean oil
Milk and dairy products
Liver

Toxicity occurs only when an overdose of vitamin K is given as a drug. An excess causes serious damage to red blood cells. Vitamin K is not included in multi-vitamin preparations, and unlike the other fat-soluble vitamins, is not stored by the body to any significant degree.

VITAMIN C (ASCORBIC ACID)

Vitamin C has many essential functions. It is involved with amino acid metabolism, hormone production, bone and tooth formation, normal growth, wound healing, and maintenance of cell membranes. It is also an antioxidant and plays a role in immune responses and allergic reactions.

Recommended Dietary Allowance: 60 mg

Much larger amounts are being advocated by some scientists, with doses up to 100 times as great as the recommended allowance. Various benefits are cited, including a lessening of cold symptoms, lowering of blood cholesterol levels, improved wound healing, protection against pollutants and environmental toxins, improved adaptation to stress, and a general bolstering of the immune system. However, studies to date have not been compelling enough to persuade the medical community, and the recommended daily allowance stands.

Man is unable to produce vitamin C in the body, nor can the vitamin be stored for any length of time. It must therefore be taken every day, either in the diet or by supplement. Overcooking destroys vitamin C. (Overcooking may consist of cooking too long, or cooking in too much water, or at too high a temperature.)

Richest sources: Green peppers
Citrus fruit
Cabbage varieties
Collard greens
Other green
vegetables
Potatoes
Tomatos

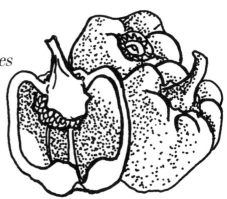

Deficiency can lead to easy bruising, bleeding gums, tissue swelling (edema), joint tenderness, increased susceptibility to infection, poor wound healing, fatigue, and ultimately scurvy, the full-blown deficiency disease, which is manifested by anemia, loosening of teeth, hemorrhages, and finally death. The description of scurvy among British sailors 250 years ago is a medical classic. Actually the condition was recognized some centuries earlier among explorers and seafarers deprived of fresh fruits and vegetables for prolonged periods. Today scurvy is most likely to occur in infants and young children sustained entirely on cow's milk.

Vitamin C toxicity is rarely encountered, even with very large doses, but massive amounts could interfere with the activity of anticoagulants (blood thinners) and vitamin B_{12}. Kidney stones have been blamed on vitamin C excess, but this connection has yet to be proved. The same goes for reports of fatigue, insomnia, nausea and diarrhea.

When a high intake of vitamin C is discontinued suddenly, the body may perceive this as a deficiency; it is a type of withdrawal effect, and could be particularly serious in a newborn whose mother took large amounts during pregnancy.

The B Vitamins

There are large numbers of B vitamins, grouped together because they were originally identified as a group. They are often found in the same sorts of food, and deficiencies, when they occur, tend to involve several of them. The eight essential Bs are thiamin, riboflavin, niacin, pyridoxine, vitamin B_{12}, folate, biotin and pantothenic acid.

THIAMIN (VITAMIN B₁)

Thiamin is water soluble and therefore not stored to any great degree. It is one of the B vitamins, required for many bodily processes, among them the metabolism of carbohydrates, and the normal functioning of the heart and nervous system.

Recommended Dietary Allowances
Men aged 19–50: 1.5 mg
Men aged 51 plus: 1.2 mg
Women aged 19–50: 1.1 mg
Women aged 51 plus: 1.0 mg

Deficiency in its full-blown form leads to beriberi, a disease that affects the heart, nerves, and muscles, and also mental functioning. Milder cases may manifest themselves with weakness, loss of appetite, constipation, pain and tingling of arms and legs, insomnia, irritability, and cardiac symptoms.

As is true for other B vitamins, thiamin deficiency rarely occurs as an isolated condition, but rather tends to be associated with other deficiencies of the B complex. This is not surprising, because many dietary sources are common to the whole group. Nevertheless, in societies that depend on white polished rice as their main staple, specific thiamin deficiency is not uncommon. Alcoholics are also at risk.

Richest sources: Whole grains
Enriched cereals
Lean meats
(especially pork)
Organ meats
Nuts
Legumes

Toxicity is not a problem because excessive amounts are excreted. Allergic reactions may occur when the vitamin is given by injection.

RIBOFLAVIN (VITAMIN B₂)

Riboflavin is one of the water soluble B vitamins. It is required for growth and metabolism; it also helps to maintain healthy skin and the linings of the digestive tract, lungs and blood vessels.

> *Recommended Dietary Allowances*
> *Men aged 19–50: 1.7 mg*
> *Men aged 51 plus: 1.4 mg*
> *Women aged 19 – 50: 1.3 mg*
> *Women aged 51 plus: 1.2 mg*

Deficiency causes sores at the angles of the mouth, skin ailments, eye problems, and personality disorders. It occurs most frequently in alcoholics, and is usually associated with other B vitamin deficiencies.

> *Richest sources: Milk and dairy products*
> *Organ meats*
> *Eggs*
> *Green vegetables*
> *Enriched cereals*
> *Bread*

Toxicity is not a problem, because only limited amounts of the vitamin are absorbed.

NIACIN (NICOTINAMIDE, NIACINAMIDE, NICOTINIC ACID, VITAMIN B₃)

Niacin is one of the water-soluble B vitamins. It plays a vital role in cell metabolism and is required for the disposition of fats and carbohydrates. It also assists in the production of some hormones. Unlike most other vitamins, niacin can be synthesized by the body if the appropriate nutrients are provided (particularly tryptophan).

Niacin differs in another way: it has functions apart from those of a vitamin. In large doses it reduces cholesterol in the blood, particularly the most undesirable fractions; such large doses, however, can have unpleasant side effects.

Recommended Dietary Allowances
Men aged 19–50: 19 mg
Men aged 51 plus: 15 mg
Women aged 19–50: 15 mg
Women aged 51 plus: 13 mg

Deficiency is most likely to occur in alcoholics and in populations whose chief food staple is corn (Mexico) or millet seed (India). It may cause skin problems, sore tongue, loss of appetite, weakness, intestinal upsets, irritability and depression. The full-blown form is known as pellagra, and is characterized by a variety of skin abnormalities, swollen painful tongue and mouth, vomiting and diarrhea, and severe mental and neurological symptoms.

Richest sources: Liver and other organ meats
Meat
Poultry and fish
Peanuts and peanut butter
Enriched cereals and breads
Green vegetables
Nuts
Legumes

In large doses nicotinic acid (but not nicotinamide) causes flushing, itching and hives, and overactivity of the intestinal tract. In sensitive individuals it may provoke an asthmatic attack.

PYRIDOXINE (VITAMIN B₆)

Pyridoxine is a water-soluble B vitamin. It is necessary for the formation of red blood cells and plays an essential role in amino acid and fatty acid metabolism. It also aids in numerous other enzyme reactions. Pyridoxine works closely with other B vitamins, and particularly contributes to the functions of niacin. Pyridoxine requirements increase on high protein diets.

Recommended Dietary Allowances
Men: 2.0 mg
Women: 1.6 mg

Deficiency is rare except in cases of alcoholism and severe malnutrition. When it occurs, it may be manifested by nausea, weight loss, anemia, sores of the skin and mouth, and nerve damage. In infants, severe deficiency may cause seizures and mental retardation.

Richest sources: *Blackstrap molasses*
Liver and other organ meats
Poultry and fish
Eggs
Whole grains
Nuts
Legumes
Bananas
Avocados

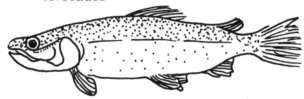

When given in supplemental doses, pyridoxine interferes with the utilization of some drugs, particularly certain medications used in epilepsy and in Parkinson's disease. Excessive doses are toxic to the nervous system, and cause numbness and tingling of the hands and feet and unsteadiness in walking. Dependency can also develop, so that rapid withdrawal of substantial doses may produce deficiency symptoms which in turn may again harm the nervous system.

VITAMIN B$_{12}$
(COBALAMIN, CYANOCOBALAMIN)

Vitamin B$_{12}$ is required for all cell production. Deficiency is displayed particularly in cells that have a rapid turnover, such as red blood cells.

Recommended Dietary Allowance: 2.0 mcg

To be utilized, this vitamin requires the presence of intrinsic factor, a substance normally elaborated by the stomach. An adequate intake of folate is also necessary. In the absence of intrinsic factor, dietary B$_{12}$ cannot be processed by the intestine and must therefore be given by injection. If this is not done, a disease called pernicious anemia will gradually manifest itself, with symptoms ranging from wide-spread damage to the nervous system to weakness, pallor, burning tongue and psychiatric problems. In the presence of intrinsic factor, B$_{12}$ deficiency does not occur, except possibly in strict vegetarians.

Richest sources: Liver and other organ meats
Egg yolks
Dairy products
Meat
Fish
Fortified cereals

Small amounts may also be produced in the small intestines.
When there is no specific deficiency of vitamin B$_{12}$ or of intrinsic factor, shots of B$_{12}$ or of liver extract serve no useful purpose.

FOLATE (FOLIC ACID, FOLACIN)

Folic acid is one of the B vitamins. It works closely with vitamin B_{12} toward normal cell production, and is particularly important during rapid growth and in pregnancy. Unlike vitamin B_{12}, folate is found in a great variety of foods, including vegetables, but it is also destroyed more easily, especially with prolonged cooking.

Recommended Dietary Allowances
> *Men: 200 mcg*
> *Women: 180 mcg*

Deficiency causes the formation of abnormal blood cells and ultimately anemia. It may be the result of poor nutrition, alcoholism, or intestinal disease, which impairs folate absorption. Unlike vitamin B_{12} deficiency, folate deficiency does not cause neurologic problems.

Richest sources: Fresh green vegetables
> *Liver and other organ meats*
> *Egg yolks*
> *Fortified cereals*
> *Legumes*
> *Bananas*

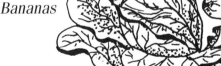

Even large doses of folate are well tolerated. Nevertheless, folic acid should not be taken casually, and particularly not for unspecified anemia, because the response to folic acid can mask the anemia caused by vitamin B_{12} deficiency, and allow neurologic damage to proceed.

BIOTIN

Biotin is one of the B vitamins. It is involved in protein, fat, and carbohydrate metabolism and may also help to maintain the texture of skin and hair.

Estimated daily requirement: 30 to 100 mcg

Deficiency is exceedingly rare, because biotin can be synthesized in the intestine. Nevertheless, it can occur with long term biotin-deficient intravenous feeding, or with the prolonged ingestion of very large quantities of raw egg white (20 or more raw eggs a day!). Excessive consumption of raw egg whites causes biotin deficiency because raw egg white contains a unique substance that binds to biotin, making it unavailable for its usual functions. Under these very rare and bizarre conditions, biotin deficiency may cause scaling of the skin, hair loss, sore tongue, muscle pain, loss of appetite, weakness and mental depression.

Richest sources: Liver and
other organ meats
Peanuts
Walnuts
Peanut butter
Egg yolks
Chocolate

Toxicity has not been demonstrated.

PANTOTHENIC ACID (PANTOTHENATE, VITAMIN B$_5$)

Pantothenic acid is one of the essential B vitamins. It is a component of enzyme systems required for the metabolism of proteins, carbohydrates and fats, for the maintenance of normal skin and internal organ linings, and for the production of some hormones. The name means "obtained from everywhere," and, true to its name, this vitamin is widely available in foods.

Estimated daily requirement: 4–7 mg

Deficiency has not been clearly demonstrated in man, although there have been reports of burning feet, headache, fatigue, and depression when a deficiency was deliberately induced. Actually even very poor diets seem to satisfy the minimum requirement.

Richest sources: Liver and other organ meats
Egg yolk
Mushrooms
Whole grains
Enriched cereals
Peanuts

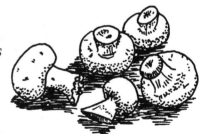

Toxicity is not known. Large doses have been taken without ill effect.

MYO-INOSITOL AND PHYTIC ACID

There are several inositols. The one usually considered in human nutrition is myo-inositol. It is present in various forms in plants and animals. In some plants, especially in cereal grains, it is in the form of phytic acid.

Extensive animal studies have been done, but in the human the significance of myo-inositol has not been fully elucidated. It appears to play a role in fat metabolism, and is reported to reduce the accumulation of cholesterol and triglycerides. It may also contribute to normal nerve conduction. Whatever its nutrient function, however, myo-inositol does not qualify as a vitamin, even though it is sometimes grouped with the B complex. Structurally it is related to glucose.

Adequate quantities are apparently produced by the body, especially in the intestine, so that it is difficult to establish a minimum need or a deficiency syndrome. The average daily intake is about 1 gm, mostly from plant foods. Inositol is often added to infant formulas, because human milk contains about three times as much as cow's milk. No deleterious effects have been reported from large supplemental doses of inositol. Excessive amounts of phytic acid, however, eaten in the form of cereal grains and grain products, may tie up some minerals, especially calcium, iron, and zinc, and interfere with their absorption. It is interesting that zinc deficiency was first described in men on high-phytate cereal grain diets.

PABA, PANGAMIC ACID, AND OTHER NON-VITAMINS

This group is the darling of salesmen and self-styled health promoters.

PABA is often grouped with the B vitamins ("B$_x$"), but by prevailing criteria it is not a vitamin in man. It is widely distributed in nature, and also produced in the intestine. There is no established requirement, and no known deficiency state or toxicity. PABA is used on the skin as a sunscreen agent. Claims that it prevents hair loss and graying of hair are not justified.

Pangamic acid is not a vitamin. It is a substance of variable composition and dubious value, touted by some as a B vitamin ("B$_{15}$") and advocated to counteract aging, heart disease, and liver damage. "Pan" means "all" and "gam" means "seed"; pangamic acid is in fact derived from seeds and from the large pits of fleshy fruits. There is no known requirement or deficiency disease. Depending on the specific ingredients, pangamic acid supplements may not be safe.

Laetrile and *amygdalin* are derived from fruit kernels and from almonds. (Amygdalin means almond.) Once called vitamin B$_{17}$ and hailed as a cancer cure, these related substances have been found ineffective, and can be toxic, because they contain a significant amount of cyanide.

"Vitamin P" consists of citrin, hesperidin, rutin, quercetin, and other flavonoids, a group of substances obtained from plants, especially citrus fruits. Claims on their behalf are numerous; these substances are said to prevent easy bruising and strokes, increase the resistance to allergies and colds, and help to reduce high blood pressure and elevated blood cholesterol. In controlled studies the claims have not been borne out. Quercetin supplements probably are not safe.

"Vitamin U" is yet another pseudovitamin, this one extracted from cabbage leaves. It has been promoted for the treatment of peptic ulcers.

FASCINATING FACTS ABOUT VITAMINS

• The term vitamin comes from the Latin *vita* (life) and denotes a substance essential for life. The word is often used loosely, however, and more than a few substances are sold as vitamins, even though there is no proven dietary need for them, and no deficiency syndrome has been demonstrated. In this group are rutin, hesperidine, bioflavonoids, pangamic acid, and PABA among others.

• The total combined weight of all eight essential B vitamins is about 31 mg per day. That means that one ounce would satisfy the needs of nine hundred people.

• Surplus vitamins do not increase energy or enhance athletic performance.

• It has never been shown that a natural vitamin is superior to a synthetic one.

CHAPTER V

Minerals, Some Essential, Some Deadly

Minerals are essential nutrients. Like vitamins, they are required in the diet for normal growth and functioning. Unlike vitamins, they are inorganic substances, that is, they are simple chemicals rather than complex carbon compounds. And unlike vitamins they are actually incorporated into cells and tissues.

Some minerals are present in the body in relatively large amounts; these are sodium, potassium, calcium, magnesium, chlorine (as chloride), phosphorus (as phosphate), and sulfur.

Other minerals are required in much smaller quantities; these are the trace elements, also known as trace minerals or micro-minerals. This group includes iron, manganese, zinc, copper, fluorine (as fluoride), iodine, selenium, chromium, cobalt, and molybdenum; all perform significant functions. There are others yet whose role is still being studied, among them boron, nickel, tin, silicon, and vanadium.

With good health the mineral levels in the blood are amazingly constant. Extra amounts are excreted; conversely, when blood levels threaten to drop, the body will deplete its own stores to maintain a steady state, such as by taking calcium out of bones. These mechanisms are delicate and complex and they can break down when the system is interfered with. Certain drugs, such as diuretics (water pills), can cause selective losses of some minerals; so can prolonged vomiting and diarrhea. The delicate balance can also be upset when excessive doses of a mineral are taken as a supplement; this can start a cascade of abnormalities affecting one or more of the other minerals and their function.

SODIUM

Sodium chloride is the combination of sodium and chlorine, known by all of us as table salt. Sodium makes up 39 percent of the salt molecule.

Salt has been prized throughout the ages. In certain times and places it was considered more valuable than gold. On the other hand, as long as four thousand years ago, Chinese medical writings warn against a high salt intake. Salt has also left its mark in many superstitions.

Salt is an essential ingredient of the human diet, but hardly in the quantities that we consume. Except under unusual conditions, we get an adequate amount of salt from a balanced diet, without ever using a salt shaker. (Even with increased salt loss, such as occurs with profuse sweating, it is generally more important to replace the water than the salt.)

Estimated daily requirement of sodium: 500 mg

This amount translates to about ¼ teaspoon of salt a day, including all the salt naturally present in food or added during processing. As can be seen from the chart below, a glass of tomato juice or a half cup of cottage cheese will just about meet the need. The average intake in the United States is 4,000 – 5,000 mg/day, almost ten times the amount needed; among some ethnic groups it is even twice that.

In the past several decades a lot of research has gone into studying the possible adverse effects of sodium. In predisposed individuals excessive salt intake seems to promote high blood pressure, or at least allow it to develop. Although a cause and effect relationship has not been proved, and other factors enter into it, it is fairly clear that high blood pressure and stroke are considerably more common in modern societies in which salt consumption is very high; the reverse is true for populations with low salt consumption.

Our taste for salt is acquired. Since excessive amounts could be harmful, it makes sense not to introduce saltiness to infants and young children in the mistaken belief that it will make food more appealing; actually it only creates an unhealthful eating pattern. We should also realize that a taste that is learned can also be unlearned, regardless of one's age!

Food labels that contain the words "sodium" or "soda" indicate that the product contains salt in one form or another. A label reading "very low sodium" means that the product contains 35 mg of salt or less per "serving" (but a serving may be smaller than usually expected). "Low sodium" means 140 mg or less per serving. The term "reduced sodium" indicates that the product contains no more than one fourth of the usual amount of salt. "No salt added" means what it says, but gives no information on the amount of sodium naturally present in the food item.

Salt substitutes usually are compounds that replace the sodium with potassium to produce a potassium salt. They are not risk free, especially when taken with some medications, or when kidney function is impaired, but they do provide a salty taste.

Three-quarters of the salt we eat is part of processed food, rather than added in cooking or at the table. Among the saltiest foods are those that are pickled, canned, smoked or cured. (Canned soup may be "good food," but it contains lots of salt.) Salty taste is definitely not a reliable indicator of the actual salt content. Ounce for ounce, for example, some dry cereals contain more salt than potato chips.

The following list gives some examples of sodium content:

Foods	Sodium (mg)
FLAVORINGS	
Table salt, 1 tsp	2,300
Soy sauce, 1 tbs	1,030
Catsup, 1 tbs	156
Mustard, 1 tbs	190
Italian salad dressing, 1 tbs	315
GRAIN PRODUCTS	
Pepperidge Farm white bread, 1 slice	123
Wonder bread, white, 1 slice	175
Saltine crackers, 3 pieces	120
Corn flakes, 1 oz	320
Cheerios, 1 oz	290
Shredded wheat, puffed rice or wheat	0
SNACKS	
Potato chips, 1 oz	210
Salted peanuts, 1 oz	138
Pretzels, 1 oz	450
LUNCH FOODS	
Bologna, 1 oz slice	285
Boiled ham, 1 oz slice	375
Dry salami, 1 oz	633
Pork sausage, 1 link, 2 oz	800
Frankfurter, 2 oz	650

Foods (continued)	**Sodium (mg)**
Tuna, canned in oil or water, 6½ oz can	910
American cheese, 1 oz slice	390
Cottage cheese, ½ cup	460
FAST FOOD	
McDonald's Big Mac	1,010
Burger King Whopper	990
CANNED SOUPS	
Black bean soup, 1 cup	1,200
Chicken noodle soup, 1 cup	1,100
Manhattan clam chowder, 1 cup	1,600
Tomato soup, 1 cup	875
BEVERAGES	
Club soda, 1 cup	55
Orange juice, 1 cup	2
Tomato juice, 1 cup	486
MISCELLANEOUS	
Dill pickle	900
Sauerkraut, ½ cup	777

POTASSIUM

Potassium is one of the major minerals in the body. It is found chiefly within cells, rather than in body fluids. Along with the other electrolytes, sodium and chloride, it helps to regulate fluid balance in the body. Potassium is also important in the transmission of nerve impulses, for the control of heart rhythm and for the smooth functioning of muscles.

Estimated daily requirement: 2,000 mg

Potassium is widely available in food, particularly unprocessed food, and deficiency does not occur under normal conditions. Prolonged vomiting or diarrhea, however, results in potassium loss. In a similar vein some diuretics (water pills), laxatives, and heart medications increase the need for potassium, and supplements may be required; these should be taken only under a physician's supervision.

Potassium deficiency is serious. It leads to muscle weakness and lethargy, and may cause heart rhythm disturbances.

Potassium is abundant in most vegetables, fruits, meat and fish. For quick or frequent feedings, bananas, orange juice, and tomato juice are good choices. Other rich sources are dried fruits, melons, nuts and peanut butter. And most salt substitutes contain a high concentration of potassium.

As with many nutrients, the human body is amazingly adept at utilizing the amount of potassium that it needs, and excreting the rest, as long as the potassium comes from food sources. In this way it is absorbed at an appropriate pace, transferred into cells, and never allowed to exceed a safe level in the circulation. (This can be said only for healthy individuals; in some conditions, particularly kidney disease, potassium intake may have to be limited.) When formulated as a medication, potassium is a potent drug that must be monitored with care.

Potassium excess is rare except with kidney disease, but when it occurs it has serious consequences. Irregular heart rhythms and abnormal heart activity are the most ominous toxic effects and require emergency treatment.

CHLORIDE

Chloride is the combining form of the element chlorine. As a component of salt (sodium chloride), it occurs naturally in numerous foods, and is also added to many of the foods we eat. Despite their close association, the requirements and concentrations of sodium and chloride differ, and the two elements function independently.

Chloride plays an important role in maintaining the delicate acid-base and fluid balance in the body. It is also a major ingredient of gastric acid, needed for digestion in the stomach.

Estimated daily requirement: 750 mg

Deficiency does not occur with any kind of reasonable diet, although prolonged vomiting or sweating may lead to depletion. Just as with sodium, most of our supply comes from processed food, and almost all the rest from the salt shaker.

CALCIUM

Of all the major minerals, calcium is the most plentiful in the human body. Ninety-nine percent of it is found in bones. During childhood, when bones and teeth are being formed, an adequate intake is particularly important. The need never stops, however, because we constantly excrete calcium and therefore must replenish it. To complicate things further, calcium is not always absorbed and utilized properly, even when adequate amounts or supplements are ingested. This is especially true as people get older. Other measures may then have to be taken to promote calcium utilization and prevent excessive calcium loss and thinning of bones. A preventive regime is best started in early middle age; any such program should be under medical supervision.

In addition to its role in bone and tooth formation, calcium is necessary for normal blood clotting, nerve and muscle function and regulation of heart rhythm. Recent studies suggest that adequate calcium intake also plays a role in preventing high blood pressure.

Recommended Dietary Allowances
Ages 19–24: 1,200 mg
Ages 25 plus: 800 mg

Deficiency may be due to inadequate intake, but other factors are more likely to be responsible. These include hormone imbalance, vitamin D deficiency, metabolic disturbances, and conditions that interfere with intestinal absorption. The symptoms and signs of low calcium levels in the blood are usually tied to the basic cause. For example, a low calcium is usually found in cases of rickets, but the primary cause for both low calcium and rickets is a vitamin D deficiency.

In the absence of serious disease, the body attempts to maintain a normal calcium level in the blood, even at the expense of drawing it out of the bones. If this mechanism proves inadequate, blood calcium levels drop and there may be muscle spasms, cramps, neurologic disturbances, and mental changes.

Richest sources: Milk and milk products
Sardines and other canned fish
Oysters
Green vegetables
Bean curd

Inordinate amounts of calcium in the diet can interfere with the absorption of other minerals and also cause constipation.

Calcium toxicity, however, is rare, because under normal conditions the body readily deals with this excess. More commonly, high calcium levels in the blood are due to other causes (just as deficiency is usually not a matter of intake alone). These causes may be hormonal or related to various disease states. Elevated calcium levels can cause abdominal upsets, weakness, and changes in behavior. Ultimately the kidneys will be damaged.

PHOSPHORUS

Phosphorus is an essential mineral, involved in numerous activities; it may in fact have more different functions than any other mineral in the body! It is a necessary component of all body tissues, required for metabolic reactions and energy production. Eighty percent of it is found in the bones and teeth.

> *Recommended Dietary Allowances*
> *Ages 19–24: 1,200 mg*
> *Ages 25 plus: 800 mg*

Deficiency is very rare, because phosphorus is widely available, particularly in protein-rich food. It may occur, however with excessive use of magnesium-aluminum antacids. With deficiency there is thinning of bone and weakness.

> *Richest sources: Eggs*
> *Milk and dairy products*
> *Meat*
> *Poultry*
> *Fish*
> *Whole grains*
> *Nuts*
> *Legumes*

Phosphorus excess can lead to calcium loss.

MAGNESIUM

Magnesium is an essential mineral, found chiefly in bone, but present in all body tissues. It is important in bone and tooth formation and for normal functioning of nerves and muscles. Magnesium is also a component of many enzymes.

> *Recommended Dietary Allowances*
> *Men: 350 mg*
> *Women: 280 mg*

Deficiency does not occur in healthy individuals on balanced diets, but it may develop in cases of alcoholism, poorly controlled diabetes, kidney disease, intestinal malabsorption, and excessive intake of phosphates. Diuretics (water pills) and prolonged intravenous feeding may also reduce magnesium.

Deficiency can lead to weakness, twitching and trembling, muscle cramps (tetany), erratic behavior and irregular heartbeat. In pregnancy, magnesium deficiency may contribute to high blood pressure.

> *Richest sources: Legumes*
> *Green vegetables*
> *Nuts*
> *Whole grains*
> *Chocolate and cocoa*
> *Seafood*

Magnesium levels may rise in some disease states, and also with the abuse of magnesium-type antacids. Excess leads to nausea, vomiting, diarrhea, and a drop in blood pressure. Ultimately respiratory failure may ensue. People with poor kidney function are especially at risk.

SULFUR

Sulfur is one of the major essential minerals, notably as a component of several amino acids, hormones, vitamins and enzymes. It is found in all tissues, with the greatest concentration in bone, hair and nails.

A daily requirement for sulfur has not been established.

Richest sources: Cheese
Eggs
Milk
Meat
Nuts
Legumes

A diet even barely adequate in protein will supply sufficient sulfur. Deficiency symptoms have not been described, and neither has toxicity from excessive amounts in the diet.

Essential Trace Minerals

These elements, though essential, are required in very small amounts; the total substance of all the trace minerals in the human body would fit into a thimble. The essential trace elements are iron, zinc, copper, manganese, iodine, fluoride, selenium, molybdenum, chromium, and possibly cobalt.

IRON

Iron is one of the trace elements. It is found chiefly in the blood as a component of hemoglobin, and is required for the transportation of oxygen to all tissues. The bone marrow, liver and spleen also contain substantial amounts of iron.

Recommended Dietary Allowances
Men: 10 mg
Women aged 19–50: 15 mg
Women aged 51 plus: 10 mg

The human body retains iron well. It has been said that unless one is losing blood, one gets enough iron by walking by a rusty pole now and then. That is almost true. Extra needs do arise when there is blood loss, or when a greater requirement is imposed by rapid growth, pregnancy, or lactation. Despite an otherwise adequate diet, women of menstruating age may get an inadequate amount of iron if their total caloric intake is modest or if they eat no animal proteins.

Richest sources: Liver
Meat
Egg yolks
Dried fruits
Fortified cereals

Deficiency leads to anemia, eventually manifested by pallor, fatigue, and decreased resistance to infection. There may be difficulty in swallowing. Nails may become malformed.

Vitamin C enhances iron utilization, and iron cookware adds a certain amount of iron to food!

Excessive iron supplementation may interfere with the absorption of zinc. In infants it can cause copper depletion. Large overdoses may be fatal in children, and adult-size supplements (which often look like candy) must be kept out of their reach.

ZINC

Zinc is one of the essential trace elements. It is a component of enzymes, bones, teeth, blood cells, testes, and several other organs. Zinc also plays a role in normal growth and sexual maturation, and is important for the healthy functioning of the immune system.

Recommended Dietary Allowances
Men: 15 mg
Women: 12 mg

Deficiency may cause loss of taste, poor appetite and fatigue. It can interfere with normal wound healing, physical growth and sexual maturation.

Richest sources: Oysters
Fish and shellfish
Organ meats
Meat
Egg yolks

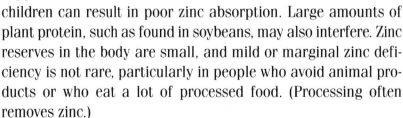

High milk consumption and high-dose iron supplementation in children can result in poor zinc absorption. Large amounts of plant protein, such as found in soybeans, may also interfere. Zinc reserves in the body are small, and mild or marginal zinc deficiency is not rare, particularly in people who avoid animal products or who eat a lot of processed food. (Processing often removes zinc.)

Low zinc levels have been reported in certain diseases, particularly rheumatoid arthritis, but a true deficiency has not been demonstrated, nor is there any proven cause-and-effect relationship. Studies are also in progress to evaluate zinc supplementation for the prevention of visual loss in the elderly.

On the other side, excessive intake of zinc is not harmless. It interferes with the availability of copper, and may thus cause anemia. It also produces gastrointestinal side effects, such as vomiting and diarrhea. As is true for many supplements, megadoses can have serious consequences. In the case of zinc, too little and too much may both have adverse effects on the immune system.

COPPER

Copper is one of the essential trace elements, found chiefly in bone, muscle, liver, and blood. It is required by the red blood cell for the proper utilization of iron in the production of hemoglobin. Copper also assists in amino acid metabolism and in enzyme formation.

Estimated daily requirement: 1.5–3.0 mg

Most people get adequate amounts of copper in their daily diet. Low copper levels are associated with protein malnutrition.

Recent studies suggest that an inadequate copper intake may lead to anemia and cholesterol elevation. Children born with a defect in copper absorption suffer from poor bone formation and retarded growth, unless the condition is recognized and treated.

Richest sources: Organ meats
Shellfish
Lean meats
Legumes
Nuts

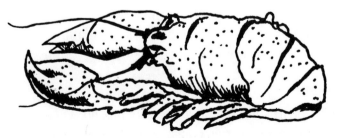

Interference with copper utilization can be brought about by large supplemental doses of zinc or megadoses of vitamin C. Inordinate copper intake is well tolerated, and symptoms of toxicity are very rare; abdominal symptoms, muscle pain, and ultimately liver damage could result from prolonged copper excess.

MANGANESE

Manganese is one of the essential trace elements. It is a component of enzymes, and plays a role in nerve function and in reproduction. It is also necessary for normal bone and tendon structure.

Estimated daily requirement: 2.0–5.0 mg

Richest sources: Whole grains
Cereal products
Peanut butter
Tea
Fruits and vegetables

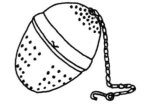

Manganese is widely distributed in plant foods.

A deficiency state has not been substantiated, but some research has suggested that inadequate manganese may play a role in osteoporosis. Manganese toxicity does not occur, even when very large amounts are eaten. Prolonged inhalation of manganese dust or fumes, however, can damage the nervous system, causing gait disturbances, tremors and slurred speech.

IODINE

Iodine is one of the essential trace elements. It is readily available in areas near the ocean, where it is found in water and soil, but the natural supply may be inadequate in inland areas. As a significant component of thyroid hormone, iodine is necessary for normal thyroid activity, which controls the body's metabolism.

Recommended Dietary Allowance: 150 mcg

Deficiency causes hypothyroidism (depressed thyroid function), which results in sluggish metabolism, fatigue, and cold intolerance. Chronic lack of iodine can produce goiter. Women who are severely deficient during pregnancy may give birth to mentally retarded children (cretins).

Richest sources: Iodized salt
Saltwater fish
Shellfish
Dairy products

Eggs, meats, and vegetables vary widely with regard to iodine content, depending on the iodine content of the soil. It is therefore recommended that people in inland areas use iodized salt. Incidentally, the iodine in milk comes mainly from the iodine disinfectants used on dairy farms!

Paradoxically, high doses of iodine also suppress the thyroid, and this facility has been used to treat overactive thyroid glands. Goiters have actually been reported in areas where iodine-rich sea weed is a major food staple. On the whole, the body adapts well to a broad range of iodine intake, and symptoms of deficiency or excess are now rarely seen in Western society.

FLUORIDE

Fluoride is the combining form of fluorine, one of the trace elements. There is some controversy about calling fluoride essential, but without much doubt it is beneficial. It contributes to firm bone structure, and is a component of tooth enamel, giving it strength and providing resistance to cavities.

Fluoride is found in almost all food and water, but not necessarily in meaningful amounts.

Estimated daily requirement: 1.5–4.0 mg

Deficiency contributes to tooth decay. In children it can also compromise the strength of bones, and in the elderly it may promote bone loss (osteoporosis).

Richest sources: Water containing adequate fluoride
Fish, especially small fish eaten with bones
Tea

For some time now there has been a heated debate about the advisability of adding fluoride to the water supply in fluoride-poor areas. Objections are based on an aversion to forced medication, and also on the fear of toxicity. Persistent and excessive intake of fluoride (fluorosis) can indeed cause mottling and pitting of teeth in children, and massive overexposure leads to kidney damage and to undue thickening and growth of bone.

In recommended doses, however, fluoridation is accepted by most scientists and health care providers as an important public health measure. One part per million (0.0001 percent) is the recommended amount in the water supply. It has been shown that the incidence of caries (cavities, tooth decay) is reduced significantly by fluoridation. Baby teeth also benefit from fluoride treatments by the dentist. Fluoride toothpaste and mouthwash may be helpful too.

SELENIUM

Selenium is one of the essential trace elements. It works closely alongside vitamin E as an antioxidant, and as such it protects against assaults attributed to free radicals. Human data for the salutory effects are not as compelling as animal data, but they seem to pertain.

Recommended Dietary Allowances
                        Men: 70 mcg
                    Women: 55 mcg

Drinking water in selenium-poor areas contains less than 1 mcg of selenium per quart. In selenium-rich areas there is up to 300 times as much.

Infants in selenium-poor areas, particularly some parts of China, have a relatively high incidence of a specific type of heart disease; this can be prevented with selenium supplementation. The only deficiency symptoms reported in adults are muscle pain and weakness after long-term intravenous feeding; this seems to respond to selenium administration.

Richest sources: Organ meats
                    Molasses
                    Grains grown in
                        selenium-rich soil
                    Fish and shellfish

When selenium intake is excessive over a prolonged period , or with occupational exposure, toxic effects may be seen. These include hair loss, nail deformities, skin eruptions, nervousness, nausea, and offensive body odor.

MOLYBDENUM

Molybdenum is one of the trace elements, considered essential because it is part of an important enzyme system. It facilitates copper and iron metabolism.

Estimated daily requirement: 75–250 mcg

Deficiency has not been described, except possibly in patients who receive nothing but intravenous feedings for a prolonged period. In such a situation it is difficult to sort out what symptoms are caused by what deficiency, but apparently molybdenum supplementation alleviates some of them.

Richest sources: Grains
Grain products
Legumes
Milk

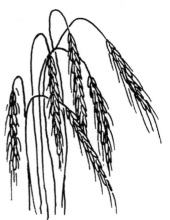

Excessive amounts of molybdenum reduce copper levels and interfere with its function. Very large doses can cause swelling of joints, similar to gout.

CHROMIUM

Chromium is one of the essential trace elements. It helps maintain normal blood sugar levels and may play a role in cholesterol metabolism.

Estimated daily requirement: 50–200 mcg

Deficiency is difficult to demonstrate, but it has been shown that diabetics on inadequate intakes improve their handling of sugar when chromium supplements are given. Patients on prolonged intravenous feedings, and the elderly, could also be subject to deficiency, and be impaired with regard to blood sugar and fat metabolism.

> *Richest sources: Liver*
> > *Clams*
> > *Peanuts and peanut butter*
> > *Grains and grain products*
> > *Corn oil*
> > *Some beers and wines*
> > *American cheese*

No toxicity has been reported from eating large amounts of chromium-rich foods. Industrial exposure, which may be hazardous, involves chromate, a compound not found in food.

COBALT

Cobalt has no known independent function, but is a necessary constituent of vitamin B_{12}. In vegetarians who depend on the small amounts of B_{12} possibly produced in the intestine, cobalt intake could be essential.

> *Estimated daily requirement: less than 1 mcg*

> *Richest sources: Fish*
> > *Peanut butter*
> > *Organ meats*

No independent deficiency symptoms have been described. Toxicity occurs only with huge doses (10,000 times the estimated need), and affects red blood cell formation and thyroid function.

TRACE ELEMENTS NOT PROVED ESSENTIAL

Boron: Although not yet included in the list of essential trace elements, boron may play an important role in bone metabolism, and could soon be acknowledged as one of the many necessary ingredients of a healthy diet. It appears to offer protection from osteoporosis, either by sparing calcium or by enhancing hormone activity when hormone levels are low—thereby promoting calcium utilization. The richest sources are fruits, cabbage, nuts, and legumes. Large doses of boron are toxic to the kidneys, and can be fatal. (Boron is toxic enough to be used as an insecticide.)

Tin: Tin is an element not known to be required by humans, but apparently needed by some animal species for normal growth. The richest sources are cereal products (bread, crackers, pasta). Prolonged storage of food in old-fashioned tin-alloy cans may allow some amount of tin to leach into the canned food product. If the amount is large, it can interfere with the absorption of zinc.

Silicon: The need for silicon in human nutrition has not been proved, but in some animal species it is required for orderly development of bones and connective tissue and also for maintenance of normal brain composition. High-fiber plants are the richest source.

Toxic effects are conceivable if trisilicate antacids are taken steadily over many years. (More hazardous is the long-term inhalation of silica dust, exposing miners and sandblasters to silicosis, a serious and potentially fatal lung condition.)

Nickel: Nickel may play a role in cell and cell membrane structure. Several animal species require nickel for normal growth and blood cell formation, but no dietary need has been demonstrated in man. The richest sources are oysters, grain products, legumes, cocoa and black pepper.

Vanadium: Vanadium is required by some animals for normal thyroid function and perhaps growth and reproduction, but it has not been proved essential in human nutrition. It is found in minute amounts in shellfish, fish, and many other foods.

TOXIC ELEMENTS

Toxic elements, many of them "heavy metals," have no proved nutritional value in man, although lead, arsenic, and cadmium, in tiny amounts, are essential in some animals. In any significant quantity they are poisonous to humans, each in a different way. Ingestion, as well as inhalation, should be avoided.

Lead: Lead is a serious health hazard, even when health effects are not obvious or acute. Until recently, the chief source of poisoning was probably lead-based paint, eaten in the form of paint chips and peelings from the walls of old buildings, or from painted cribs and other furniture. With public education and legislation regarding paint composition, headway has been made toward prevention.

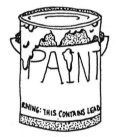

Drinking water is now receiving some of the attention it deserves with regard to lead content. Lead contamination may come from the water source itself, or from pipes made of lead or soldered with lead. Five parts per billion is considered the maximum acceptable lead level; it is significantly higher in many places. (Historians have said that the Roman empire fell because lead poisoning from lead water pipes was so prevalent. This is not likely, because it is known that the Romans were well aware of the hazards of lead plumbing.)

There are several more insidious sources of toxic lead: vegetables grown in soil that is contaminated by the remains of previous buildings, soil itself, if it is eaten in the form of clay or putty (a practice not uncommon in some areas), old china, particularly if the glaze has been worn away by time or dishwasher detergent, and food from old tin cans that were soldered with lead. Lead inhalation is also hazardous. This includes persistent exposure to leaded gasoline or the lead dust generated in many industries.

The effects of lead poisoning are usually gradual and cumulative. Lead is particularly dangerous to infants and young children, and also to pregnant women, because they transfer lead to the fetus. In children, it causes mental retardation and delayed physical development. Other toxic manifestations, which can occur in adults too, are loss of appetite, anemia, irritability, weakness, high blood pressure, hearing loss, and kidney damage. Some of these effects are irreversible.

It may require a blood test and a little detective work to diagnose lead poisoning. Once the suspicion has been raised, particularly regarding the water supply, the problem should be checked out. Tests are readily available from government and commercial sources. Most local health departments will cooperate fully, especially when the health of children is involved.

Mercury: Mercurial waste materials and fungicides may contaminate fish and agricultural products. The source of the mercury is not always clear; it may be the result of direct industrial pollution, but it may also come from emissions or dumping some distance away.

Chronic poisoning results in metallic taste, loss of appetite, anemia, kidney damage, irritability, visual problems, tremors, spasticity, mental aberrations, and, in children, mental retardation.

Mercury contained in dental fillings (amalgam) has not been

shown to pose a health hazard in humans. Small amounts of mercury apparently do escape from such fillings and may be deposited in body organs, but the amounts are evidently too small to cause demonstrable disease.

Arsenic: Tiny quantities of arsenic are required by some animal species, and trace amounts may someday prove to be essential in the human diet.

Before the advent of antibiotics, arsenic was used in the treatment of many diseases, including syphilis and tuberculosis. On the other hand, because it is tasteless, arsenic has also been a favorite poison for many centuries. Aside from the acute effects (often death), chronic poisoning from various medications and nostrums was not rare. Nowadays toxic effects may result from contamination by herbicides and fertilizers. Symptoms include diarrhea, garlic odor of breath and sweat, darkening of the skin (especially eyelids), disturbed sensations, loss of appetite and weakness; ultimately there is liver and kidney failure.

Cadmium: The use of cadmium in industry has increased over the past few decades, and with this increase some cadmium has entered the food chain through contamination of water and soil. When ingested by grazing animals, cadmium is concentrated in the liver and kidneys; the organ meats of deer and moose particularly should be avoided.

Smokers can absorb cadmium from cigarette smoke. Paint and galvanized pipes have also been impugned. Although the amounts that are absorbed are usually small, cadmium settles in the tissues, and over the years can damage the kidneys and other organs. It has been suggested that cadmium exposure also contributes to hypertension.

Radon: Radon is a radioactive gas that occurs naturally in the soil in many areas. When trapped in an enclosed space—such as a house built on contaminated ground—radon is a health hazard on the ground floor, especially to the lungs. Radon levels can be tested fairly easily; many inexpensive EPA-tested detection kits are available. The presence of small quantities of radon can be countered with rather simple measures.

Aluminum: Although often accused, aluminum utensils and cookware have never been shown to cause any damage. The debate continues, however, about other aluminum sources, in particular water. Since abnormal aluminum deposits are found in the brains of patients with Alzheimer's disease, a relationship is being sought between high aluminum levels in the local water supply and the incidence of this disease, but the verdict is still out.

Aluminum antacids are another possible source of aluminum.

FASCINATING FACTS ABOUT MINERALS

• Sea water contains 3.5 percent salt, or almost half a tablespoon of salt per 8 ounce glass—not as much as soy sauce, but more than almost any other food item. Even fish can't drink sea water. They either process it or obtain the necessary water from the food they eat, be it animal or vegetable.

• Even unbalanced diets are likely to supply the essential minerals in adequate amounts, with two exceptions. One is iodine; in deficient areas this must be remedied with iodized salt. The other is iron, frequently deficient in premenopausal women.

• Three minerals, sodium, potassium, and chloride, comprise the major electrolytes; that means that among other tasks it is largely their responsibility to maintain the acid-alkali and water balance in the blood. The balance is very critical and must be precise; even small shifts can cause major problems; large shifts threaten life itself.

CHAPTER VI
Familiar Subjects

W e take it for granted that we know a lot about these topics. We deal with most of them every day. Nevertheless, closer examination may reveal some of the finer points.

NUTRIENTS

Nutrients are defined as essential components of the human diet. All the substances listed below must be present. Anything not mentioned is not a dietary requirement.

Water.

Proteins: These must include the essential amino acids: isoleucine, leucine, lysine, methionine, phenylalanine, threonine, tryptophan, valine, and, especially in infants, histidine.

Carbohydrates: These include sugars, starches, and cellulose (fiber).

Fats: These must include the two essential fatty acids, linoleic acid and linolenic acid; arachidonic acid is also essential, but can be produced by the body, provided that adequate amounts of linoleic acid are present.

Vitamins: These include the fat soluble A, D, E, and K; and the water soluble C and eight Bs—thiamine, riboflavin, niacin, pyridoxine, vitamin B_{12}, folate, biotin and pantothenic acid.

Minerals: These include sodium, potassium, chloride, calcium, phosphorus, magnesium, sulfur, iron,. zinc, copper, manganese, iodine, fluoride, selenium, molybdenum, chromium, and possibly cobalt.

Water, cellulose, vitamins, and minerals contribute no calories to the diet. Protein, sugar, and starch, in pure form, provide about 4 calories per gram and are therefore equal with regard to food energy. Fats provide 9 calories per gram and, weight for weight, are thereby more than twice as fattening.

WATER

It provides no calories, and may not always be to everyone's taste, but water is one nutrient we cannot live without. There is no cell, tissue, or organ that does not require water for normal functioning. Life as we know it cannot exist in its absence.

Our bodies are one-half to two-thirds water; in a 150-pound individual, that's about 10 gallons! Depending on body size, activity, dietary factors, and climate, the daily turnover is usually between two and four quarts. In hot weather, with exercise, as much as 15 quarts may be lost in a day. Too much water (within reason) is readily excreted, but an inadequate intake is hazardous, and can be more rapidly fatal than the lack of any other nutrient.

Water is obtained from food as well as from liquids. Some

foods, especially fruits and vegetables, have a very high water content; peaches, pears, oranges, and apples are up to 85 or 90 percent water; green beans, peppers, lettuces, cabbages, squashes, and several other vegetables have an even higher water content. In an average diet, at least a third of the water we consume comes from "solid" food.

The excretion of water is handled mainly by the kidneys in the form of urine, but water is also lost as sweat through the skin, in the air exhaled through the lungs, and in the stool.

Water varies widely in mineral content. "Soft" water is relatively mineral-free; it makes nice suds and leaves little deposit. "Hard" or mineral-rich water is often tastier, and may or may not be better for your health, depending on the minerals in it. As a rule, if a water softener is to be installed, it is best to attach it only to the hot water pipes, which supply water for bathing and laundry, and leave the minerals in the cold water for drinking, cooking, and outdoor chores.

Water must be monitored regularly, regardless of its source, because it may contain disease causing bacteria and chemical pollutants (arsenic, benzene, nitrates, nitrites, lead and radioactive substances). Boiling kills bacteria, but does not remove chemicals. Even distilled water may not be entirely pure; it also tends to be tasteless.

Bottled water, usually obtained from springs, contains varying amounts of minerals. When the concentration of minerals is above a certain level, it is considered a "mineral water," whether the mineral content is natural, or adjusted by the bottler. Similarly, in sparkling water, the carbonation (carbon dioxide gas) may come from a spring or may be introduced by the company.

Bottled water has become big business, partly for reasons of taste, but partly also because some consumers don't trust their water supply. Springs, however, can be contaminated and polluted, just like other water sources, and must be monitored regularly.

A large industry has sprung up around home water purification. Several systems are in common use. Reverse osmosis machines and high-volume carbon filters remove many contaminants, but bacteria and some toxic chemicals may remain. Faucet filters are usually inadequate. When safety, rather than taste, is a concern, it is best to rely on the findings of an independent lab (mail-order if necessary), or on data from the local utility company, rather than on information provided by a company that sells purification equipment.

MILK

A great variety of milks is available to consumers. The following outline gives some of the types, and their characteristics.

Whole milk: cow's milk that contains a minimum of 3.25 percent milk fat (butter fat), and a minimum of 8.25 percent non-fat milk solids.

Homogenized milk: milk that has been pumped under pressure through tiny holes of a homogenizer; the process reduces the size of fat globules and maintains an even distribution of the fat throughout the liquid.

Pasteurized milk: milk that has been heated to 145 degrees for 30 minutes or to 158 degrees for 15 seconds; this destroys most organisms, particularly disease-causing bacteria and fungi.

Ultrapasteurized milk: milk that has been heated well above the boiling point (but without boiling), for two or more seconds; this is a form of pasteurization, and it also increases the milk's shelf life.

Acidophilus milk: whole milk to which bacteria have been added that help digest lactose.

Raw milk: unpasteurized, unprocessed milk. Because of the danger of bacterial contamination, raw milk is considered unsafe and is banned by many states. Some states permit raw milk if it is produced and certified by supervised dairies.

Low-fat milk: pasteurized milk whose fat content has been reduced to 1 or 2 percent. The percentage is marked on the container.

Skim or non-fat milk: milk whose fat content has been reduced to less than a half percent.

Evaporated milk: ultrapasteurized homogenized whole milk from which about 60 percent of the water has been removed.

Evaporated skim milk: skim milk with about 60 percent of the water removed.

Condensed sweetened milk: evaporated milk combined with a quantity of sugar, usually sucrose.

Dry (powdered) whole milk: pasteurized whole milk from which all water has been removed.

Non-fat dry (powdered) milk: pasteurized skim milk from which all water has been removed.

Cultured buttermilk: pasteurized low-fat milk in which bacteria have been cultured to create the characteristic taste.

Imitation milk: milk from which all milk fat has been removed and replaced by other fats or oils, in order to minimize cholesterol content. The product may contain highly saturated oils.

Human milk (breast milk): Ounce for ounce, human milk has slightly less protein and more carbohydrates, fat, and calories

than cow's milk. It contains considerably less vitamin D than fortified cow's milk or commercial soy formulas. Quite uniquely,
about 10 percent of the unsaturated fatty acids in breast milk are
of the omega-3 variety.

Human milk contains several other substances lacking or
deficient in cow's milk. Some, such as choline, inositol and taurine
are now being added to infant formulas. Others, for example
carnitine, are being studied and considered for addition. Breast
milk possibly imparts to the infant a degree of protection against
some infectious diseases and allergies. It can also transfer
substances which are not desirable and may be hazardous.
Narcotics, tranquilizers, alcohol, nicotine, and many medications,
including some antibiotics and laxatives, are excreted in breast
milk and may affect the nursing infant.

Soybean-based infant formula and soybean milk: soybean
products used when milk is to be avoided for reasons of digestive
problems, allergy or vegetarianism.

Goat milk: usually not pasteurized, not licensed, not safe. It
has a higher fat content and more calories than cow's milk.

Lactose: the sugar naturally present in the milk of mammals.

Casein: milk protein, a standard for measuring the nutrient
characteristics of other proteins.

CALORIE AND FAT CALORIE CONTENT OF
DIFFERENT MILK VARIETIES

	Calories (per 8 oz)	Calories from Fat (per 8 oz)
Whole milk	150	72
homogenized		
pasteurized		
ultrapasteurized		
raw		
reconstituted dry whole milk		
imitation milk		
Low-fat milk, 2 percent	121	42
Low-fat milk, 1 percent	102	23
Cultured buttermilk	100	20
Skim or non-fat milk	86	2
Half & Half	324	255
Light cream	504	445
Heavy cream	835	806
Evaporated whole milk	338	171
Evaporated skim milk	200	7
Condensed sweetened milk	980	238
Human milk	180	94
Goat milk	168	91
Soybean-based infant formula (avg)	165	80
Liquid non-dairy creamer (avg)	320	215

ALCOHOL

References to alcohol are found in some of our earliest records. Then as now, alcohol was used for medicinal and ritual purposes, as well as for its pleasurable effects. Most fruits and grains and many vegetables were found to be fermentable, and spirits of all sorts were produced. Nevertheless, excessive use of alcohol is frowned upon by almost all societies; some religions forbid it entirely.

Alcohol provides calories, but has no other nutritive value. By displacing food in the diet, reducing appetite, disturbing digestion and metabolism, and through toxic effects on the liver it may cause malnutrition in chronic heavy users and ultimately lead to serious illness.

Although alcohol in all its forms is a central nervous system depressant, it is initially perceived to be a stimulant, because it first tends to depress an individual's inhibitory centers, thus lessening tension and allowing for more relaxed behavior and communication. At the same time, mood control and judgment are actually impaired, and there is an escalating loss of mental and physical abilities as the blood alcohol level rises.

Generally speaking, the "stronger" the drink, the more calories per ounce of liquor. Mixers, while diluting the strength per ounce, may add calories to the whole.

A can of beer, five ounces of table wine, and a jigger (1 ½ oz) of straight liquor have about the same intoxicating effect, but beer has the most calories. Light beer has fewer calories than regular beer, but the alcohol content is about the same. The following list compares (approximately) various representative alcoholic drinks with regard to calories and alcohol content.

	Amount (oz)	Calories	Alcohol (gm)
GIN, VODKA, WHISKEY, RUM			
80-proof	1½	104	15
100-proof	1½	125	18
LIQUEURS (cordials)	1	100	7
BRANDY, COGNAC	1	70	10
COCKTAILS			
Manhattan	3½	165	20
Martini	3½	140	19
Daiquiri	3½	131	15
Old-fashioned	4	180	24
WINES			
Table, red or white	5	105	13
Champagne	5	106	14
Aperitif (dry sherry)	2	85	9
Dessert (port)	3½	135	16
BEER			
Standard	12	150	13
Light beer	12	95	13

Alcohol blood levels serve to confirm alcohol consumption and to determine the degree of intoxication. The following guidelines may be used:

Percentage of Blood Alcohol	State of Intoxication
.00 to .04	You have been drinking.
.05 to .09	You may be drunk.
.10 to .14	You are drunk.
.15 and higher	You are dead-drunk.

For the purpose of defining "driving while intoxicated" (DWI), most states accept 0.09 percent as the legal upper limit of acceptable blood alcohol. On the average, the body is able to metabolize about 10 grams of pure alcohol, or slightly less than an ounce of 80 proof whiskey, in an hour. The speed of drinking, therefore, plays a role in the degree of intoxication. Non-alcoholic men are able to dispose of alcohol more readily than women or than chronic alcoholics of either sex.

For a gross estimate of blood alcohol levels, the following chart may be used. It is based on body weight and on the amount of alcohol consumed on an empty stomach in a one-hour period.

BLOOD ALCOHOL LEVELS
(percent alcohol in blood)

Gin (oz)	Wine (oz)	Beer (cans)	Body Weight					
			120 lb	140 lb	160 lb	180 lb	200 lb	220 lb
2	7	1½	.07	.06	.05	.04	.04	.03
3	10	2	.10	.09	.08	.07	.06	.05
4	13	3	.13	.12	.10	.09	.08	.07
5	17	3	.17	.14	.13	.11	.10	.09
6	20	4	>.20	.17	.15	.13	.12	.11
7	23	5		>.20	.18	.16	.14	.13
8	27	5			>.20	.18	.16	.15
9	30	6				>.20	.18	.17
10	33	7					>.20	.19
11	37	7						>.20

Note: > = more than.

CAFFEINE

Coffee plants have been grown for their stimulative properties for over a thousand years. Coffee is a newcomer, however, when compared to tea which has been cultivated for at least 3,000, and possibly 5,000 years. Both arrived in Europe in the seventeenth century, coffee from the Middle East and tea from the Far East.

Caffeine, the active ingredient in both beverages, is a drug. Its stimulant properties are real. It promotes alertness and counteracts fatigue; thinking becomes clearer, and manual skills are improved. In most adults the stimulant effects are mild and pleasurable. In children and in sensitive individuals, or when taken in excess, there may be adverse effects on the heart and nervous system, manifested by rapid or irregular heart-beat, trembling, anxiety, and insomnia. Some of these effects can carry over to the unborn fetus or the breast-feeding infant; pregnant and lactating women should therefore limit their coffee intake.

Detractors claim that coffee increases cancer risk, causes fibrocystic breast disease, infertility and birth defects, raises cholesterol, and leads to high blood pressure. None of this has ever been found true in humans, although adverse effects have been observed in laboratory animals on very high doses of caffeine.

Coffee may aggravate ulcer symptoms. This is equally true for decaffeinated coffee; obviously, gastric irritants other than caffeine are involved. All types of coffee and tea should be avoided if they cause gastrointestinal problems.

Excessive doses of caffeine cause jitteriness, disturbances of heart rhythm, insomnia and dehydration. Caffeine is addictive. In habitual users caffeine is needed for normal functioning. When it is stopped abruptly, withdrawal symptoms may occur for several days, manifested by mental and physical sluggishness, headache and irritability.

Listed below are ranges of caffeine content in some common products. The exact amount varies with different methods of manufacture and preparation.

Beverages	Caffeine (mg)
Coffee, 5 oz	60 — 180
Tea, 5 oz	20 — 110
Decaffeinated coffee or tea, 5 oz	1 — 5
Hot cocoa, 5 oz	4 — 25
Chocolate milk, 8 oz	2 — 7
Cola drinks, 12 oz	30 — 50
Diet colas, 12 oz	30 — 50
Decaffeinated cola drinks, 12 oz	1 — 10

Foods	
Baking chocolate, 1 oz	25 — 35
Dark chocolate, 1 oz	5 — 35
Milk chocolate, 1 oz	1 — 15
Chocolate syrup, 1 oz	5

Drugs (per standard dose)	
Anacin	64
Excedrin	130
No Doz	200
Vanquish	66
Vivarin	200

TOBACCO

Tobacco was introduced to Europe by Columbus's crew on their return from the New World; from there it spread rapidly to all the other continents. Despite the compelling evidence of the detrimental consequences of smoking, billions of people throughout the world continue to smoke. In the United States alone, 1.5 billion cigarettes are sold daily.

The addictive component of tobacco is nicotine, which affects the central nervous system. As with other addictive substances, tolerance is rapidly built up in the beginning; and when the drug is stopped the user experiences withdrawal symptoms. It was thought at one time that cigarette smoking is not "addicting," but rather habit-forming and a type of compulsive behavior like overeating. This is not true; the dependence is physiological as well as psychological.

Regardless of the way it is taken, by smoking, chewing, or intravenous administration, nicotine produces a feeling of well-being in the regular user; it is actually calming and stimulating at the same time. Withdrawal causes anxiety, irritability, and difficulty in concentrating.

The addictive nature of nicotine is, however, almost the least hazardous effect of cigarette smoking. The great damage comes from the burning of tobacco, which releases tars, carbon monoxide and, in all, several *thousand* unwelcome substances. Many of these substances affect not only the smoker, but also other people in the environment. Heart attacks, emphysema, stroke, cancer of the lung, lip, tongue, and esophagus . . . these are just a few of the conditions caused or facilitated by the use of tobacco.

Cigarette smoking is the greatest *preventable* cause of death and illness in our time. The cigarettes the United States exports to cocaine-producing countries kill more people in those countries than does the cocaine they send to us.

CHAPTER VII
Safety Issues and Controversies

U nlike the previous chapters, which deal with established information, some topics in this group are likely to provoke strong differences of opinion. Still, it is worthwhile to separate facts from myths to the best of our ability.

ORGANIC FOOD

The health food industry and its customers use the term "organic" to denote produce that was grown without chemical fertilizers or pesticides. Unless it is certified by a supervising agency, however, there is no guarantee that the claim is valid. Different states define "organic" differently. Some require a minimum of three years between the last chemical application and the time of harvest. Others allow the term "organic," but set no guidelines on time. More than half the states are not concerned with definitions at all and set no rules.

Organic produce may be two or three times as expensive as its supermarket counterpart. The same is true for meat from animals that were raised "organically"—that is, with no chemicals by injection or in the feed.

Chemical fertilizers, when properly constituted and applied, are generally not a health hazard. A plant ordinarily will extract from the soil the nutrients it needs, whether these are provided by manure or by chemicals. As a matter of fact, artificial fertilizer can sometimes be tailor-made to supply a mineral or other substance in which that particular soil is deficient. When properly managed, organically and non-organically fertilized plants have the same nutritional value, taste, and appearance. This does not mean, however, that the unrestrained use of chemicals should be permitted. Plants can and do pick up unwanted substances when they are present in excess; and aside from damaging the produce, these chemicals can also kill wildlife and pollute the water tables. Pesticides, fungicides, and preservatives are an even more serious concern. They adhere to plant surfaces and may intrude into the plant itself.

Most organic growers do, in fact, avoid the use of chemicals —fertilizers, pesticides, herbicides, fungicides, fumigants—but one would almost have to farm on virgin territory, in a remote part of the world, not to be affected by chemical contaminants to some degree, whether these are brought in by wind or water, or left behind from previous treatments.

The terms "organic" and "natural," when applied to meat and poultry, promise a product free of antibiotics and hormones. Hormones are used to promote growth and composition, and to provide a faster and larger yield. As in the case of chemical fertilizers, hormones are almost certainly harmless when used responsibly and in measured amounts. But is supervision adequate?

At this point the consumer must judge the evidence and make the decision. Theoretically at least, there is no denying the appeal of organic farming. Whether it can succeed in an environment of industrial pollution and acid rain is questionable. And it is even more questionable whether it can produce maximum amounts of food in a world that must deal with famines, depleted soil, and vanishing farmland.

"HEALTH FOODS," "HEALTH FOOD" SUPPLEMENTS, AND "NATURAL FOODS"

Over the past several decades we have made great strides in the science of nutrition, and the public has become much more aware of the importance of a healthful diet. For a variety of reasons there is also a growing tendency toward self-diagnosis and self-treatment. Unfortunately, along with this burgeoning interest, increasing numbers of self-styled nutrition experts and health food promoters have come on the scene, many with fancy (though meaningless) titles and degrees, and most of them more skilled in salesmanship and oratory than in science. They stage today's sophisticated version of the medicine show, and their wares are today's snake oil.

All of us want to eat foods that promote good health, but some foods and supplements make more sense than others.

Alfalfa, important as animal fodder, is promoted for its mineral, vitamin, and chlorophyll content. It is however largely indigestible by humans.

Bee pollen is the tiny male seed found in blossoms. The commercial product may also contain nectar (plant secretions) and bee saliva. Bee pollen has been advocated as a treatment for sterility, hardening of the arteries , poor muscle tone, etc., etc. These claims have never been substantiated by any scientific studies. Undeniably bee pollen contains amino acids, vitamins, and minerals, but it is a very expensive source of nutrients that are readily available elsewhere.

Bioflavonoids: see flavonoids.

Bone meal is a mineral supplement that features large doses of calcium and other components of crushed or ground-up bone. It is not recommended, because the product often contains unwanted contaminants, including lead.

Brewer's yeast (debittered, non-leavening yeast) can serve as a source of B vitamins, amino acids, and minerals, but it offers no advantage over other foods that contain these nutrients. One tablespoon has about 25 calories.

Carob is obtained from the pod of a Mediterranean tree. It is used as a substitute for chocolate, because it has less fat and is free of stimulants. Incorporated in a candy bar, however, it is combined with other ingredients, and ends up with a fat and calorie content similar to chocolate.

Chlorophyll plays an important role in plant metabolism, but serves no nutritional function in humans. It is promoted as an internal deodorant.

DNA and **RNA**, ribonucleic acids, are specific and integral components of all cells, both animal and vegetable. Supplements, however, are not utilized and are useless.

Dolomite is a mineral supplement derived from limestone. It is rich in calcium and magnesium, but measurements are not accurate or dependable. Dolomite may also include hazardous impurities, such as lead.

Flavonoids (or *bioflavonoids*) are substances found in plant foods, chiefly in the rinds; they are reputed to supplement the actions of vitamin C. *Hesperidin,* from citrus fruit, and *rutin,* usually from buckwheat, are the best known among them. Along with *Acerola C,* a berry, and *rose hips,* the nodules under rose buds, they are variously grouped together as vitamin C complex or vitamin P. Bioflavonoids can also be derived from algae. Notwithstanding the claims, flavonoids have not been shown to play a role in human nutrition.

Garlic, an ancient folk remedy, believed to ward off disease as well as vampires, may in fact have beneficial health effects. There is no hard evidence so far, but garlic and its many components are being studied for possible medicinal properties.

Ginseng is a Chinese herb whose root is reputed to have the power to restore natural balance and sexual potency. Ginseng can cause an increase in blood pressure, diarrhea, nervousness, and insomnia. Its hormonal effects can be damaging to the unborn fetus, and the use of ginseng is most inadvisable during pregnancy.

Granola is a tasty non-specific combination of ingredients, among them oats, wheat germ, honey, brown sugar, coconut, raisins, nuts, seeds, and spices. It is usually high in calories and fat. Depending on the exact composition, a cup of granola can provide over 500 calories, half of which may come from fat.

Honey is probably the oldest cultivated sweetener, loved throughout the ages. Except for some minerals, present in very small amounts, honey offers no nutritional advantage over table sugar, especially in the quantities that are ordinarily used.

Kelp is a supplement produced from seaweed. It is a rich source of iodine and also of magnesium and calcium. It may also contain harmful amounts of arsenic.

Macrobiotics are various cereal grains. A true macrobiotic diet is nutritionally incomplete. (Macrobiosis actually means "longevity," but long life is not furthered by a deficient diet.)

Megavitamins are very large doses of vitamins, with amounts far greater than required for good nutrition. Some megavitamins are useless, but harmless; some are toxic, particularly megadoses of vitamins A and D; and some, while not toxic in themselves, may interfere with the utilization of other nutrients. Since vitamins are used by the body in trace amounts, mega doses don't make sense. If a serious vitamin deficiency exists, or if one seeks a specific medicinal effect of a vitamin, this should be handled under a physician's care. As long as minimum needs are met, extra vitamins do not provide extra energy or protection from illness.

Natural is not a meaningful term when applied to food, because there are no standards of definition. And being natural doesn't necessarily make a substance desirable in one's food.

Papain (papase) is an enzyme found in papaya. Because it breaks down protein, it is used to tenderize tough cuts of meat, but it does little when taken as a tablet.

Royal jelly is a substance secreted by worker bees to promote the development of the queen bee. It does nothing for human beings.

Vegetarianism that permits eggs and dairy products (lacto-ovo vegetarianism) allows for an adequate protein intake, but may be high in saturated fat and cholesterol. Strict vegetarians who avoid all animal products must be circumspect about getting enough protein and vitamin B_{12}.

Vitamin B_{12} injections are worthless in healthy individuals who eat a balanced diet.

Wheat germ, a portion of the wheat seed, is a rich source of vitamin E. It also supplies some minerals and B vitamins. An ounce of toasted wheat germ has 108 calories, 25 percent of them from fat.

HERBS AND HERBAL TEAS, ROOTS AND BARKS

Starting with the most ancient civilizations, herbs have been known for their medicinal properties. Our oldest written document, the Ebers papyrus, 3500 years old, contains a description of herbal treatments. Many subsequent cultures produced elaborate and comprehensive herbals, and some present-day societies still depend on the healing powers of herbs.

Many plants do indeed have potent medicinal properties, among them foxglove, belladonna, and henbane. In most instances the active ingredients have been identified and can now be synthesized. Manufactured drugs are safer than extracts of medicinal plants: they can be produced without impurities, they are uniform and of predictable strength, and they are subjected to extensive testing and quality controls.

Herbal teas pose a related problem. They are promoted for being natural products (so are coffee and tea!), and for being free of stimulants. Some herbal teas, in fact, do contain significant amounts of caffeine. More important, they can be health hazards in several ways: medicinal ingredients in the tea can produce unexpected and undesirable effects; the herbs may have been sprayed or contaminated with toxic chemicals (supervision is poor); and allergic reactions are not uncommon (chamomile, for instance, is related to ragweed). Unless marketed by a reputable company, herbal teas are best avoided.

There are literally thousands of plants that have been used for medicinal or mystical reasons. Some with truly dangerous potential are classified as poisonous plants. Mentioned here, alphabetically, are some of the better known herbs, roots, barks, etc., all available in stores or by mail order. They can be harmful, particularly when given to the very young or old, when taken in excess, or when used in place of conventional medicine to treat an illness.

Here is a selection:

HERBS, ROOTS & BARKS
Promoted as Health Foods

achuma	elecampane	licorice
aconite	euphorbia	ma hueng
akee	eyebright	mohudu
aloe vera	fritilleria	monkshood
astralagus	gentian	pau d'arco
baneberry	ginkgo leaf	polygala tenuifolia
biloba	ginseng (see	probolis
black cohosh	Health Foods)	quassia
burdock root	golden seal	saffron
cananga	gotu-kola	sarsaperilla
castor	guarana	schizandra
catnip	hellebore	skullcap
chamomile	ho shou wu	snake root
chickweed	hyssop	soksi
comfrey	iboga	spirulina (an alga)
culebra	Iceland moss	squaw vine
damiana	ipe roxo	taheebo
dandelion	jojoba	thistle
dong quai	kava kava	valerian
echinacea	lantana	yarrow

FREE RADICALS AND ANTIOXIDANTS

Free radicals are the extra unpaired electrons found on some molecules. Such a molecule becomes very active, trying to find another molecule to which the electron can attach itself. Not only will this damage the new-found molecule, but it can start a chain reaction, as the new unbalanced molecule seeks yet another recipient.

Oxygen radicals are the most common culprits. They can be found in the environment, in food, and within our bodies as the result of normal reactions. The healthy organism can usually rid itself of these radicals, but even the healthiest may not be able to deal with a massive assault, such as that produced by heavy X-radiation. Air pollution, smoking, pesticides, viruses, chemicals, improper food storage and handling (heating fats too hot or too often), and unfiltered sunlight have all been implicated in the formation of free radicals. Free radicals are suspected of playing a role in the causation of many disorders: cancer, hardening of the arteries, autoimmune diseases such as rheumatoid arthritis and lupus, and possibly Alzheimer's disease and the whole aging process.

Antioxidants, by definition, delay or prevent oxidation, blocking free oxygen radicals, and rendering them harmless as it were. This protects tissues from damage.

Vitamins A, C, and E and selenium are the nutrients believed to have significant antioxidant activity. Other nutrients and several drugs are being studied for their antioxidant properties.

Specific groups of people may be more in need of antioxidants than others. Smokers require extra amounts of vitamin C; consumers of large amounts of unsaturated fatty acids need more vitamin E; and people exposed to drugs, chemicals, and environ mental pollutants may *also* benefit from added antioxidants. The field is far from being fully understood.

IRRADIATION OF FOOD

Food irradiation is a very effective method of combatting some serious agricultural problems: the bacterial contamination of poultry and seafood, the insect infestation of grains, nuts and spices, and the sprouting and too rapid ripening of vegetables and fruits. Irradiation is not used much, however, because its full effects have not been established with certainty, and the public is wary, if not downright opposed to the concept. The process is also very expensive.

The main objections to irradiation are safety issues: the possible changes within the molecules of the food stuff, particularly the creation of free radicals, and the destruction of vitamins. There is also the fear that resistant bacteria might survive and flourish. In any event, viruses will not be eliminated, and neither will toxins that were produced by bacteria prior to irradiation (the toxin that produces botulism, for example). Some opponents also suggest that irradiation might be used as a substitute for cleanliness and meticulous processing.

On the other side, it must be said that no apparent harm came to astronauts or to American troops in Vietnam who ate irradiated meals, and no untoward effects have ever been demonstrated in animals given irradiated feed. What's more, some alternative substances or methods used to increase shelf life—such as various chemicals, insecticides, preservatives, or intense heat—carry their own adverse potentials.

Fresh food preserved by irradiation can survive long shipments and storage under less than perfect conditions. This could be a boon at times of natural catastrophe and in areas of malnutrition or famine.

Since 1958 the FDA has classified irradiation as a food additive. Under that heading its use must be approved for a specific food product, and it must be marked with the radiation logo, a circle containing a flower with a dot above it. If, however, only an ingredient has been irradiated (such as the mushrooms used for canned mushroom soup), this fact need not be disclosed.

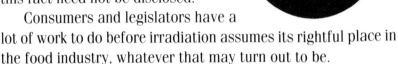

Consumers and legislators have a lot of work to do before irradiation assumes its rightful place in the food industry, whatever that may turn out to be.

ADDITIVES

Natural and synthetic substances are added to foods for a variety of reasons. Some prevent spoilage and thereby add to the longevity of a product. Some maintain consistency and texture. Some add flavor, some add color, and some even improve the nutritional value by preventing vitamin loss.

Some additives must be listed on the label (nitrites,sulfites, tartrazine, etc.), some can be lumped together ("artificial colors and flavors"), and some don't have to be mentioned at all. In general, additives must be listed if they could be unsafe under certain conditions.

Many additives are used to prolong the shelf life of food products, but they also work in the consumer's interest. They inhibit mold formation on bread, and ice crystal formation in ice cream; they keep salt from caking and cake from tasting stale.

The list of additives in our food is almost endless; the number is actually in the thousands. We rely heavily on governmental agencies to oversee their use, and on consumer groups to press for continued testing. The FDA is entrusted with monitoring all additives with a computerized program called ARMS (Adverse Reaction Monitoring System).

Coloring agents could be considered frivolous additives because they are used primarily to make food look more appealing. Without them, many consumers would miss the pale yellow of butter and margarine, the dark caramel of cola drinks, and the pretty pink of strawberry ice cream. Consumers also associate the expected color with good quality; for example, oranges that look green are often considered unripe or inferior, even though that is not necessarily the case; for this reason, oranges are often colored orange.

"Certified colors" are manufactured and each batch is tested. Coloring agents that are derived from natural products, such as carrot oil or grape juice, need not be certified. Certified (synthetic) colors are often preferred because they do not impart a flavor of their own; they are also more stable and more versatile in achieving color gradations.

Preservatives keep foods from spoiling and also from tasting stale or rancid. Salt is the oldest and still the most commonly used preservative, particularly for meat and fish. Wherever refrigeration is not available, heavy salting is still being used.

Well known among preservatives are *nitrites:* they not only preserve processed meats, but also intensify their color (bacon, hot dogs etc). Although the body actually produces its own nitrites from nitrates in the diet (nitrates are abundant in vegetables), their safety has been questioned repeatedly, because under certain conditions nitrites react to form nitrosamines which are implicated in the development of some cancers. All in all, nitrite-rich foods are best limited, or avoided when there is a choice, especially by children.

Sulfites are another group of compounds involved in controversy. Starting with the Romans, who used sulfites to cleanse their wine containers, these substances have served to inhibit bacterial growth and delay deterioration of foods. In our day, however, their main use is often for appearance; when sprayed on fruits and vegetables, sulfites make these foods look fresh and attractive—even after prolonged exposure to air. This specific use of sulfites has now been banned in salad bars, because in sensitive individuals sulfites can produce serious symptoms, including wheezing, rash, abdominal cramps, vomiting, and fainting. Salad bars are not a good idea anyway: there is too much opportunity for contamination. Wine, beer, dried fruits, seafoods, instant potatoes, soups and many other processed foods and drugs must be labelled with regard to sulfite content, so that sensitive individuals can avoid them. Wine bottled before 1988 will not be marked. Neither, of course, is restaurant food.

Sulfites are actually antioxidants, substances that protect foods from the specific hazards of oxygen, such as occurs with exposure to air. Other preservatives in this group are BHA and BHT; they too have been questioned with regard to safety. Antioxidants as a group are discussed elsewhere.

Humectants hold moisture and protect foods from drying out.

Anti-caking agents absorb moisture and allow powdered food to flow freely.

Emulsifiers keep substances mixed and uniform, even substances that normally don't mix at all, such as oil and water. Glycerides and lecithin are common examples. Emulsifiers are used in such products as salad dressings, peanut butter, and ice cream.

Sequestrants and **chelators** prevent substances, especially tiny amounts of metals, from mixing or interacting with foods, thereby spoiling or discoloring them.

Thickeners enhance the texture of such foods as yogurt and ice cream. Various gums and starches are commonly used.

Stabilizers prevent physical changes in ingredients, most notably the deterioration of flavors.

Flavor enhancers "bring out the flavor" in food. The chief one is MSG (monosodium glutamate), a substance used widely in commercial food processing. Many people report unpleasant side effects from MSG— the "Chinese restaurant syndrome"—but others deny that such a syndrome exists. MSG contains a lot of sodium (salt). Summing up: MSG should be used sparingly and should best be avoided by young children.

Fortifiers are substances not normally present in a food product that are added to improve the nutrient value. The fortification of milk with vitamin D has had a major impact on the health of children. Most additions, however, increase the cost of a product without adding significantly to good nutrition.

PESTICIDES

In any discussion of food safety, the subject of pesticides is bound to be raised as an important issue. Broadly speaking the term pesticide denotes any material that is used to control insects, molds, diseases, and weeds. Almost a billion pounds of chemicals are used annually in the United States for this purpose.

The application of pesticides is intended to enhance the quality and quantity of farm products. Unfortunately, some chemicals are pervasive; not only do they coat the fruit or vegetable, but under some conditions they may enter the product itself, and no amount of washing will remove them. Even the surfaces cannot always be cleaned effectively if the produce has been waxed, or coated with a chemical for the sake of appearance or preservation.

Nor does pervasiveness apply just to the produce for whose benefit it was intended! Chemical residue can be detected in meat, poultry, and fish, if these animals consumed pesticide-tainted vegetation. Even chemicals used on non-edible crops such as cotton, can eventually pollute the water table and enter the food chain. And some pesticides stay around for a long time: DDT residue is still found in some crops, eighteen years after it was banned!

So much for the bad news.

Chemical pesticides fulfill a need, particularly when food has to be mass-produced at reasonable cost. Insect plagues can destroy entire crops, and even milder infestations make food unacceptable. The fear of chemicals might be allayed if consumers could be sure that there is rigid control of their use, strong legislation, adequate funding, and constant monitoring.

Some progress has been made in these areas: the public has become much more educated and vocal, and several government agencies are committed to the safe and effective use of chemicals in agriculture, chief among them the Environmental Protection Agency (EPA). The Food and Drug Administration (FDA) and the U.S. Department of Agriculture also play specific roles. Nevertheless there are still rough edges in monitoring pesticide residue. Imported products are especially difficult to control since only spot checks can be done. Foreign growers may not only apply more pesticides, but they could be using chemicals not even permitted in the United States.

Fortunately, newer and safer means of pest control are being studied and developed. One technique is the use of pheromones, the scents normally elaborated by female insects to attract males; these scents can be synthesized and placed in strategic areas to confuse the males and prevent reproduction. Another trick lies in cultivating insect breeds that are harmless to food plants but feed off the harmful insects.

Promising new methods have come about through the science

of genetic engineering. The testing of a genetically engineered virus was recently approved. Bacteria and bacterial products are already in use against some beetles, larvae, and fungi. A natural virus actually has been used in farming for half a century, but it is not specific enough, and can do damage to other plants. Specificity is very important in genetic engineering. The aim is to create *specific* biological products that will be the natural enemies of *specific* pests, while being totally safe for man.

Genetic engineering may also succeed in producing crops that are more disease and pest resistant than their ancestors, and plants that can tolerate weed killers and other chemicals without damage to themselves or potential toxicity to the consumer. This is also one of the aims of scientific hybridization.

Without much doubt, chemicals will continue to be used, but here too there will be an increasing emphasis on specificity: using small amounts of the right stuff at the right time and place. Right now, less than 3 percent of all farmers in the United States farm entirely without the use of chemicals. Some farmers are actually discouraged from introducing better methods, such as crop rotation, because they are boxed into growing federally supported crops—wheat, corn, soybeans, and cotton—or lose their subsidies.

Consumer issues aside, chemical pesticides pose a particularly great hazard to farm workers. Migrant workers often live near pesticide-treated fields, along with their families, and safety rules are not always strictly enforced. Added to poor nutrition and poor sanitation, exposure to toxic chemicals makes migrant farm workers the highest risk group with regard to occupational illness.

HORMONES

Hormones are essential substances produced and secreted by specific glands of the body. Hormone-producing glands are known as ductless or endocrine glands, because they discharge their products directly into the blood stream, in contrast to exocrine glands which deliver their material to nearby areas, often by way of ducts—tears, saliva, sweat, etc.

The endocrine glands are the pituitary, thyroid, parathyroid, and adrenal glands, the sex glands—testes and ovaries—and the pancreas, which also plays an exocrine role.

Hormones serve vital functions with regard to metabolism, growth, sexual development, reproduction, and response to exercise and stress. For specific medical problems hormonal substances are prescribed; among these hormones are insulin, birth control pills, cortisone, and thyroid hormone.

Anabolic steroids ("steroids"), sometimes used and abused by athletes for muscle building, are a form of male sex hormone. An informal survey of football players showed that 10 to 25 percent of them had taken steroids. The percentage is undoubtedly even higher, particularly in some other sports, such as weight lifting. Steroids do build muscle tissue, but they also have serious side effects, possibly permanent,including liver damage, premature heart disease, sexual disfunction, aggressive behavior and other psychological problems. In women they also produce acne, male type hair growth and hair loss, and deepening of the voice.

Growth hormone, a pituitary hormone, has also been used for muscle building, primarily because it is harder to detect than anabolic steroids. Unlike steroids, it may do more for the size of muscles than for their strength. Growth hormone is a valuable drug when used for the right reasons, but muscle building for athletic performance is not one of them.

As long as nutrition is not grossly impaired, such as in starvation or with extreme weight loss, and as long as there is an adequate source of iodine, hormone production is generally not affected by specific food intake. Contrary to what some people believe, obesity is very rarely due to a hormonal imbalance. It is in fact more likely to be the other way around: morbid obesity can cause hormone imbalance; the same is true for excessive leanness sometimes seen in runners.

The injection of hormones or its addition to the feed of livestock and poultry is quite a different problem. The practice has been espoused by some, and severely criticized by others. Hormones and hormone-releasing substances can indeed enhance the quality and quantity of meat, making it leaner and promoting faster growth. Milk production can also be increased. Such practices have major economic consequences. Consumers, however, are less concerned with farm economics than with safety issues. Despite well-founded assurances by scientists and government agencies, uncertainties remain in the minds of the public about the use of hormones, particularly since the practice is usually not disclosed on the marketed product.

CARNITINE (L-CARNITINE)

L-carnitine, once known as "vitamin B_T" and "B_T factor," is a substance normally present in liver and muscle tissue. It is not a vitamin, but plays a significant role in the transport of fatty acids. Beyond infancy, carnitine is supplied by the average diet, and is also synthesized from amino acids. Newborns, however, cannot synthesize sufficient amounts, and may become deficient if fed an unfortified soy formula.

Richest sources: Red meat
Milk—including powdered and skim milk

Deficiency is very rare, but may occur as a genetic disease, and also with severe protein malnutrition, prolonged intravenous feeding or kidney dialysis. It is manifested by progressive muscle weakness.

L-carnitine is mentioned in this section because it has been promoted to athletes under the mistaken notion that it enhances energy and endurance by mobilizing fat from tissues. Some athletes are persuaded that it will substitute for steroids, and do less harm. While there has been some research that shows carnitine to increase the walking distance in individuals with very poor circulation, there is no such evidence in any controlled studies with normal people. Long-term effects of L-carnitine supplements are not known.

FOOD ALLERGIES

Food allergies most often manifest themselves with skin symptoms; sometimes the primary effect is on the respiratory or gastrointestinal tract.

When the gastrointestinal tract is the primary target, allergy must be distinguished from food intolerance, such as an inability to digest milk, and from diseases of the intestinal tract. Symptoms with all these conditions may include cramps, nausea, vomiting, and diarrhea.

When allergy affects the skin, it can produce a rash, hives, puffiness, and itching. Respiratory symptoms include sneezing, wheezing, congestion, and runny nose. Full-blown asthmatic attacks may occur. The foods most often responsible for allergy are eggs, milk, shellfish, peanuts, nuts, wheat, soybeans and chocolate. Elimination diets serve to make a diagnosis.

FOOD POISONS

Proper food handling and food storage are the best prevention against food poisoning, even though we cannot always control all the variables.

It should be routine to wash fruits and vegetables thoroughly to remove insecticides, fungicides and any other chemicals that may have been applied to the surface. A dilute solution of mild liquid soap is more effective than plain water.

Viruses, bacteria, and parasites actually produce far more illness than chemicals. The most common bacteria to cause food-related illness are salmonella and campylobacter. Chicken and other poultry should always be washed, inside and out, and so should the surfaces that meat or fish have touched. Stuffing should be added just before cooking, because stuffing provides a good growth medium for bacteria from the poultry.

Bacterial and, in some instances, parasitic infestation can occur in raw animal products. Much as we may enjoy steak tartare, sashimi, seviche, sushi, eggnog and Caesar salad, we must realize that eating raw meat, fish, and eggs carries a certain risk which is eliminated by cooking, or sometimes by prior freezing. The most hazardous foods of all are raw or undercooked oysters and clams.

Increasingly we also hear about toxic chemical contamination, particularly of fish, with substances such as dioxin and mercury; this is a problem that neither cooking nor freezing will solve.

Some foods tell you that they are no longer safe, by their odor or change in appearance; consider them inedible. Bulging or leaking cans and cracked containers should be discarded without a taste test. Food that has been sitting out on a buffet table for hours is best avoided, as is perishable food on a summer camping trip when there is no refrigeration. In fact, in warm weather it is even a good idea to bring a cooler to the supermarket, when the trip home is a very long one.

Of all the safety measures over which we have control, perhaps the simplest one is hand washing, particularly before eating.

Food poisoning should always be reported to the local Health Department if the suspected source is a processed food product or public eating place.

POISONOUS PLANTS

Poisoning from house and garden plants is not uncommon, especially among toddlers and young children. No one should taste any leaves, flowers, or berries, unless the plant is known to be safe. A poison control center should be called, when there is even a question about an unknown substance.

Eating poisonous plants can cause a variety of reactions, ranging from mild irritation in and around the mouth to severe illness that may involve almost every organ system.

Only non-foods are listed below (some under several different names). It should be remembered, however, that even common food plants can be toxic if the wrong part of the plant is consumed; potato sprouts are a prime example. Everyone knows, of course, that some mushrooms are extremely poisonous; their identification should never be left to amateurs.

Poisonous Houseplants

Caladium	Ivy	Oleander
Dieffenbachia	Jerusalem cherry	Philodendron
Elephant ear	Mistletoe	Poinsettia
Holly	Monstera	

Poisonous Bulbs

Amaryllis	Daffodil	Iris
Crocus	Hyacinth	Narcissus
Narcissus		

Poisonous Shrubs, Herbs, and Weeds

Absinth	High John root	Richweed
Aesculus	Hog's bean	Saint Bennet's herb
Apple of Peru	Horse chestnut	Saint Johnswort
Arnica	Hyoscyamus	Sanguinaria
Asthma weed	Hypericum	Scoparius
Belladonna	Irish broom	Scotch broom
Bittersweet	Jalap	Snakeroot
Bloodroot	Jimson weed	Spartium
Broom	Klamath weed	Spindle tree
Broomtop	Leopard's bane	Spotted cowbane
Buckeye	Lily of the valley	Stamonium
Burning bush	Lobelia	Sweet cane
Calamus	Madderwort	Sweet cinnamon
Conium	Mandragora	Sweet flag
Convallaria	Mandrake	Sweet root
Datura	May apple	Thornapple
Devil's apple	May lily	Tobacco
Devil's eye	Mingwort	Tolguacha
Dulcamara	Mistletoe	Tonka bean
Emetic Weed	Morning-glory	Umbrella plant
Euonymus	Mugwort	Vinca
Fool's Parsley	Nightshade*	Wolf's bane
Goatweed	Periwinkle	Wormwood
Hemlock	Podophyllum	Yohimbe
Henbane	Red puccoon	

---

* Some nightshade plants should be excepted from this list—potatoes, tomatoes, peppers, and eggplants among them. They are age-old important food crops. Nevertheless, rumors resurface or persist that they have deleterious effects, and some people avoid them.

CHAPTER VIII

Miscellaneous Topics

A s the heading says, this chapter deals with odds and ends, all connected with food in one way or another.

ENZYMES

Enzymes, defined as "organic catalysts," are substances that expedite chemical reactions in the body, without participating in the actual process. Innumerable different enzymes are needed for the innumerable processes that take place. With some exceptions, enzymes cannot be eaten. Specific body cells must produce specific enzymes for specific functions.

Digestive enzymes, secreted in the mouth, stomach, pancreas and intestinal tract aid in the breakdown of the food we eat. Other enzymes help to convert sugars, fats, and amino acids into an appropriate form for energy use, tissue development, or storage. Enzymes play a role in nerve transmission, clotting, wound healing, and drug utilization—in fact, in almost every bodily activity.

LACTASE

Lactase is an enzyme normally found in the small intestine of mammals. It aids in the digestion of milk, specifically by breaking down lactose (milk sugar) into simpler sugars (glucose and galactose) that are suitable for absorption. Most humans, as well as other mammals, lose lactase activity as they grow into adulthood, and with it the ability to digest milk. The loss is much greater in some ethnic groups than in others; evolutionary factors may play a role in this difference, since societies with a prominent dairy agriculture have a better genetic makeup for handling milk.

Ethnic Group	Approximate Percentage of Adults Affected by Lactase Deficiency
Northern Europeans	10
Mediterranean Europeans	75
Jews	80
Blacks	80
American Indians	80
Orientals	95
World population as a whole	70

Judged by mammalian standards, lactase deficiency is actually the more normal condition, because few adult animals drink milk. But, although growing up usually results in an intolerance to lactose, the deficiency is rarely complete, so that most people can tolerate small amounts of milk without discomfort; about 10 percent of the population, however, is sensitive to even the smallest quantities.

Milk chocolate, skim milk, low fat milk, whole milk, and buttermilk (in that order) are most likely to cause difficulties. Yogurt, although high in lactose, contains an enzyme in its culture that aids in lactose digestion, so that symptoms are less common and less severe. (This is not true of frozen yogurt, because freezing destroys this enzyme.) The various other dairy products are rarely a problem. One would have to eat 10 ounces of processed cheese, or a stick of butter, or a cup of sour cream to consume the lactose found in 8 ounces of milk.

Symptoms of intolerance, when they occur, may variously consist of bloating, abdominal rumbling, cramps, nausea, flatulence, and diarrhea. The most effective way of avoiding discomfort is to limit lactose intake to one's tolerance level. When taken with a meal, milk is less likely to cause symptoms than when drunk by itself. For those who want to increase their milk intake beyond tolerance, commercial lactase is available. This may be taken along with the dairy product, or it may be added to the milk some hours ahead of time so that the lactose is predigested.

To avoid any possible confusion, it should be stated that lactase deficiency is quite different from a congenital and much more serious enzyme disorder, galactosemia, which precludes the normal metabolism of galactose, and which must be treated by avoidance of all dairy products and all foods and drugs containing even the smallest amounts of lactose.

TYRAMINE

Tyramine is a derivative of the amino acid tyrosine. Its significance lies chiefly in the effect it has on individuals who are taking monoamine oxidase (MAO) inhibitors, a group of drugs at times prescribed for depression or hypertension (high blood pressure). When a patient receives such a medication and then eats one of the tyramine-rich foods, severe and possibly life-threatening reactions may occur.

Listed on the following page are foods and beverages that

contain significant amounts of tyramine:

- *Aged cheeses,* such as brie, camembert, roquefort, stilton, blue, parmesan, Swiss and cheddar (Cream cheese and cottage cheese are safe.)

- *Pickled, smoked and dried fish*
- *Smoked sausages*, such as salami, bologna, pepperoni
- *Liver*
- *Brewer's yeast*
- *Bananas*, especially green bananas
- *Fava beans* (Italian broad beans)
- *Avocado*
- *Yogurt*
- *Soy sauce*
- *Vanilla* (except in minute amounts)
- *Wine*, especially chianti and sherry, but others as well
- *Beer and ale*
- *Chocolate*

TAURINE

Taurine, a type of amino acid, participates in many metabolic processes. It plays a role in the formation of bile salts (the name "taurine" refers to ox bile) and also seems to be involved in activities of the heart and other organs under nervous control. Because the body can synthesize it from other amino acids, taurine is not considered essential in the diet.

Richest sources: Raw clams and oysters
Human milk

It is interesting that breast milk, particularly in the early months of lactation, contains large amount of taurine; cow's milk, perhaps because it is not early milk, is much lower. By the same token, formula-fed babies, especially premature infants, have lower taurine levels than breast-fed babies. Even at low levels, however, no deficiency effects have been demonstrated. Nevertheless, taurine is now being added to infant formulas, and consideration is being given to adding it to long-term intravenous feedings, particularly for infants.

ASH — ALKALINE AND ACID

The expressions acid ash and alkaline ash refer to the effect of a particular food on the acidity or alkalinity of urine after the food item has been metabolized. This is generally of importance only when it influences the effectiveness of a drug; some drugs require a certain acidity to produced their desired effect on the urinary tract.

Interestingly, some foods we consider as acid tend to make the urine more alkaline: citrus fruits are an example.

Acid-ash foods include: meat, poultry, fish, shellfish, eggs, cheese, bread, pasta, cereal, cranberries and plums.

Alkaline-ash foods include: milk and dairy products (except cheese), almost all fruits, most vegetables, corn, legumes, nuts, coffee, and tea.

KOSHER PRACTICES

Kosher means fitting or "proper." Kosher dietary laws (laws of
kashrut) concern themselves not only with food, but also with
utensils and the conduct of a meal. Here are some of the
principles:

Meat and poultry must be obtained from kosher sources,
where slaughtering, handling, and processing are supervised.

Meat must come from cloven-hoofed animals that chew their
cud (Leviticus 11:3—*Whatsoever parteth the hoof, and is cloven-
footed, and cheweth the cud, among the beasts, that shall ye eat).*
There must be no visible traces of blood; meat must be well done
(Genesis 9:4—*But flesh with the life thereof, which is the blood
thereof, shall ye not eat*; and Leviticus 17:10—*I will even set my
face against that soul that eateth blood, and will cut him off from
among his people).*

Only fish that have fins and scales may be eaten. Shellfish is
not permitted (Leviticus 11:12—*Whatsoever hath no fins nor
scales in the waters, that shall be an abomination unto you).*

Dairy products and meat may not be eaten at the same meal
(Exodus 23:19—*Thou shalt not seethe a kid in his mother's milk).*
Meat may follow a dairy food, but several hours must elapse after
a meat course before a milk product may be eaten. Separate
utensils must be used to prepare and serve meat and dairy foods.

Fish, eggs, fruits, vegetables, grains, coffee, tea, and non-
dairy fats and creamers are neutral (*parve*) and may be taken at
any time.

Passover is a Jewish religious holiday that commemorates the
Jews' exodus from Egypt. The observance of Passover requires
entirely separate sets of utensils and special dietary observances,
particularly the omission and removal of any leavened grain or
grain product, such as bread or pasta (Exodus 13:7—*and there
shall no leavened bread be seen with thee, neither shall there be*

leaven seen with thee in all thy quarters).

Kosher commercial products bear a K label or a U inside an O. These symbols represent certification by two different rabbinical organizations.

 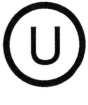

CLEAR LIQUID, LIQUID, AND SOFT DIETS

A clear liquid diet is used when solid or semi-solid foods cannot be tolerated, and when all solid matter must be withheld, even in puréed or liquid suspension form. The following items are allowed: water, apple juice, fat-free broth, bouillon, plain gelatin desserts, fruit ice, tea, and carbonated drinks.

A liquid or full liquid diet is used as a transition between the very restrictive clear liquid diet and a more permissive menu. It also serves people who have difficulty with biting and chewing. In addition to clear liquids, permitted foods include all fruit and vegetable juices, strained cream soups, milk and milk drinks, smooth cooked cereals such as farina, plain yogurt, sherbet, ice cream, smooth pudding, and custard.

A soft diet, sometimes required after surgery or for gastrointestinal or dental problems, adds the following: puréed fruits and vegetables, mashed potato, apple sauce, bananas, puréed or finely chopped meat or fowl, cream sauce, gravy, eggs, cottage cheese, butter, margarine, creamy peanut butter, refined white bread, cooked refined cereal and coffee.

CHAPTER IX

Taking Measure

M easuring, weighing, reading, interpreting—ultimately we must learn the system, and judge for ourselves, preferably with the facts in hand.

LABELS

It is important to read and understand labels, both for *what they say* and for *what they don't say.*

Ingredients arc listed in order of weight. If a frozen dinner is called "Gravy and Turkey," or lists these contents in that order, it means that the product contains more gravy than turkey. If a breakfast cereal names sugar as its first ingredient, it contains more sugar than cereal grain. Sugars may be listed by specific type, however, so the total amount is not always obvious. Nabisco Fruit Wheats, for example, lists sugar, high fructose corn syrup, brown sugar, corn syrup, and dextrose among the first eight ingredients.

If a label waffles on ingredients, assume the worst possibility. For example, soybean and/or coconut oil could mean *all* coconut oil, which is very highly saturated. The term "vegetable oil" is also vague; it too could include or consist of tropical oils.

Fats are usually listed in grams or percent of total weight, but not in calories or percentage of total calories. For example, a package of turkey bologna may read "85 percent fat free," and the ingredient list confirms this; calculations will quickly show, however, what this means, namely that over 60 percent of the total calories come from fat.*

The terms "light" and "lite" generally refer to texture or taste, and not to calorie or fat content.

There is truth in all this labeling, but it is nevertheless misleading to many consumers. Equally misleading can be the portion size found on a product label. Spaghetti, for example, lists its nutritional ingredients for two ounce servings. This is not a realistic amount for most spaghetti eaters.

Sometimes claims are made which don't mean much. A cereal advertised as containing three times as much calcium as a competing brand, or three times as much vitamin D, offers no significant advantage if the difference lies between 6 percent and 2 percent of the daily requirement.

Ingredients need not be given for products whose contents are standardized by law, such as mayonnaise. If there is a major variance, the term "imitation" has to be used, or an entirely new name can be applied (Miracle Whip). Ingredients must always be listed when a special nutritional claim is made, such as "90 percent fat free" or "low cholesterol" or "low salt."

In 1990, a new law was passed requiring nutrition information on almost all labels; the law probably will be implemented by 1993, and will cover packaged food products. Not only will nutrients be listed, but carbohydrates will specify fiber and

---

* An ounce (28 gm) of this product provides 60 calories; it contains 15 percent fat, or 4.2 gm. At nine calories per gram, 9 times 4.2 comes to 38 calories of fat, which is 63 percent of total calories. (Caloric values are described in the section on calories.)

complex carbohydrate content, and, under fats, saturated fats and cholesterol will be itemized.

When an actual health claim is made (for example, "lowers cholesterol"), the effectiveness of the product will have to be proved to the FDA with scientific testing; right now, the rules are vague.

To be called a *"dietary supplement"* a product must provide at least half of the recommended allowances of vitamins and minerals.

The term *"fortified"* means that something not normally found in the food has been added to it; a good example is milk fortified with vitamin D. The term *"enriched"* means that some ingredient that was lost during processing has been put back; an example is flour, enriched with B vitamins.

Animal products that carry a USDA label have gone through a Department of Agriculture inspection for safety. Unfortunately there are not always enough inspectors to do a thorough job. Labels marked "Prime," "Choice," or "Select" concern themselves with taste quality, not freshness or nutritional value. For this type of labeling the meat to be judged is selected by the meat-packing company. "Prime," the tastiest grade of beef, is usually highly "marbled"; it may indeed be tastier and more tender than leaner cuts, but it contains more fat, and, by current thinking, is nutritionally inferior.

To be marked "lean," meat can contain no more than 10 percent fat by weight; "extra lean" means 5 percent. The fat allowances for ground meat are more generous; they are usually described on the label.

Diet foods require careful label reading. "Sugarless" or "sugar free" indicates the absence of table sugar, but does not promise lower calories. Neither does "dietetic" mean a reduction in calories. When marked "low calorie," a food may contain no more than 40 calories per "portion," but the portion is often found to be small. "Reduced calories" must show one-third fewer calories than the original. "Low cholesterol" means no more than 20 mg per serving.

Specific additives, flavors, and coloring agents need not be listed separately, unless they are known to have caused adverse reactions in susceptible individuals or they are considered foods (onions, celery, etc).

Substances administered to animals or added to any food before it is processed by the manufacturer need not be declared. This includes antibiotics and hormones given to livestock and poultry, and preservatives that may have been used before the food went to the processor.

Net weight includes everything inside the container: the syrup of canned fruit, the oil in the sardine can, the liquid in a jar of olives.

Dates on food products cannot be understood unless the type of dating is specified. The date may indicate when the product was packed, or the last recommended sell date (which usually allows for a few extra storage days at home), or the estimated final date on which the food can be considered wholesome and fresh-tasting. Some dates are in code and cannot be deciphered by the consumer at all. This is particularly true of canned foods, whose shelf life is long, but certainly not infinite.

RDA   (Recommended Daily Dietary Allowance) is the estimated daily nutritional requirement, as formulated and published by the National Research Council. (Values quoted in this volume apply to healthy non-pregnant adults only. Recommendations for children and pregnant or lactating women should be made by a physician.)

GRAS stands for "generally recognized as safe." It is
used by the Food and Drug Administration (FDA)
to permit the unrestricted use of certain additives.

UPC (Universal Product Code) is the patch of lines and
numbers that serves as a code for food and non-
food products, and can be scanned at checkout
counters for product identification and price.

"Natural" and "organic" are not always well-defined terms,
and can be used and misused to mean many things. They are not
stamps of good nutritional quality.

CALORIES

As applied to living organisms, calories are a measure of energy:
the energy taken in as food, and the energy expended by activities and bodily processes.

Caloric requirements vary greatly, depending on age, size,
and energy expenditure. A small sedentary elderly woman may
need 1,000 calories daily, a large young man doing heavy labor
may utilize three or four times that much. Proteins, carbohydrates, and fats are the three groups of caloric nutrients.
Proteins and carbohydrates, in their pure form, provide 4 calories
per gram, or 113 calories per ounce. Fats contribute 9 calories
per gram, or 255 calories per ounce.

Quantity of Food That Supplies About 100 Calories

DAIRY PRODUCTS
Whole milk	5 oz
Skim milk	9 oz
Butter	1 tbs
Cheddar and other hard cheese	1 oz
Low-fat cottage cheese (2%)	½ cup
Low-fat yogurt	⅔ cup
Ice cream	⅓ cup

SPREADS
Oleo	1 tbs
Mayonnaise	1 tbs
Peanut butter	1 tbs
Honey	1½ tbs

MEAT, POULTRY, SEAFOOD (cooked without fat)
Sirloin steak	1½ oz
Turkey, white meat	2 oz
Cod	3½ oz
Shrimp	10 medium

CEREALS AND CEREAL PRODUCTS
Oatmeal, cream of wheat or rice	¾ cup
Wheaties, cornflakes, Special K	1 cup
Shredded wheat	1¼ biscuits
Spaghetti, cooked	½ cup

(continued)
Quantity of Food That Supplies About 100 Calories

VEGETABLES
Celery	12 stalks
Lettuce, shredded	12 cups
Tomato	2 large
Onions, chopped	1½ cups
Green beans, broccoli, cooked	2½ cups
Potato, baked	1 medium
Potatoes, french fried	7 pieces

FRUITS
Apple	1 medium-large
Banana	1 medium
Cherries	20
Grapefruit	1 large
Grapes	18–30
Orange	1 large

SNACKS
Potato chips	9 pieces
Saltines	8 pieces
Dry roasted peanuts	⅔ oz
Jelly beans	15 pieces
Chocolate chip cookies	2 pieces

BEVERAGES
Orange juice	7 oz
Cola drink	8 oz
Whiskey	1½ oz
Table wine	5 oz
Beer	8 oz

ACTIVITY AND CALORIES

Larger people will spend 100 calories more quickly; smaller people will take longer. In other words, more energy is expended for the same task by a large person than by a small one.

The figures given below indicate the approximate number of minutes that it would take a 150-pound individual to work off 100 calories. It takes the expenditure of thirty times that much to achieve a one-pound weight loss!

Nevertheless, even though moderate exercise doesn't make up for overeating, a steady regime of exercise does have an effect on weight. Two hundred *extra* calories expended each day for a year will produce an easy weight loss of twenty pounds.

TIME NECESSARY TO EXPEND 100 CALORIES

Minutes	Activity
85	Sleeping or resting
60	Sitting, quietly occupied (reading, watching TV)
36	Driving
28	Strolling (3 miles per hour)
20	Walking, moderate speed (3½ miles per hour)
17	Bicycling, moderate speed
19	Social dancing
13	Tennis
10	Jogging
9	Swimming
7	Running, 8-minute mile
5	Racing: track, bicycle or swimming

Physical activity is important for the maintenance of good health. The activity may consist of housework, child care, farm labor, or recreational exercise. Preferably it should involve several muscle groups, and at times be vigorous enough to raise the pulse rate.

FASCINATING FACTS ABOUT CALORIES

• "Diet," "dietetic," and "low calorie" on a label means that a portion may provide at most 40 calories per serving. The size of the serving, however, is left to the manufacturer's discretion, and may be smaller than expected.

• Calories are all-important in weight loss diets. Fad diets come and go, but it's the calories that count. There are tricks to eating fewer calories (less fat, fewer courses, smaller portions, no seconds), but the method that is *not* recommended is a grossly unbalanced diet. Not only can it cause adverse metabolic effects, but it cannot be maintained over the long haul, and it certainly does not promote good eating habits.

• It pays to be a calorie counter, and not be fooled by popular myth. A cup of creamed cottage cheese has about the same calories as a cup of cooked spaghetti (plain, of course). A cup of low fat fruit yogurt has more calories than a lightly buttered English muffin. A glass of orange juice has more calories than the same amount of Coke. An ounce of raisins has more calories than an ounce of jelly beans.

• Substituting 6 ounces of fish for 6 ounces of steak once a week will save over 16,000 calories a year. Switching from a cup of whole milk to skim milk every day will reduce annual calories by more than 23,000. Making sandwiches with turkey breast meat or lean ham instead of bologna or Swiss cheese twice a week results in 17,000 fewer calories. These changes are not only better nutritionally, but, added up, will result in a weight loss of almost 20 pounds over the year.

BODY WEIGHT

Many methods have been devised for determining ideal body weight. For several decades, the Metropolitan Life Insurance tables have been used as a standard. Although useful, they may be flawed in several ways:

(1) No allowances are made for age; people normally gain a modest amount of weight as they get older.

(2) Great variation is allowed for body types; for example, the "desirable" weight of a 5'4" woman can be anything from 114 to 146 pounds. While it is true that some people have larger frames than others, self-assessment is often fallacious; accurate frame analysis is rarely done. and heavy people tend to attribute their overweight to large frames.

(3) The tables are based largely on the longevity of policy holders; since people often lose weight when they are chronically or terminally ill, the statistics may unduly associate low body weight with high mortality; this factor would produce a higher ideal weight.

(4) Because of the prevalent mix of policy holders, the data are based mostly on middle-class people.

In recent years, tables have been devised that do not differentiate between men and women or body types, but concern themselves only with height and age. Other tables use only height and gender. Some tables aim for extreme leanness. Clearly there is no perfect formula for the perfect weight. Shown on the opposite page is a table with reasonable criteria. (Weight includes light clothing. Height is measured without shoes.)

Desirable Weights in Pounds

Height	Age 20–29	30–39	40–49	50–59	60–plus	Avg. U.S.
			WOMEN			
4'10	97	102	106	109	111	122
4'11	100	105	109	112	114	
5'	103	108	112	115	117	127
5'1	106	111	115	118	120	
5'2	109	114	118	121	123	132
5'3	112	117	121	124	126	
5'4	115	120	124	127	129	137
5'5	118	123	127	130	132	
5'6	121	126	130	133	135	142
5'7	124	129	133	136	138	
5'8	127	132	136	139	141	147
5'9	130	135	139	142	144	
5'10	133	138	142	145	147	152
			MEN			
5'2	121	125	126	127	126	142
5'3	125	129	130	131	130	
5'4	129	133	134	135	134	154
5'5	133	137	138	139	138	
5'6	137	141	143	144	143	166
5'7	141	145	147	148	147	
5'8	145	149	151	152	151	178
5'9	149	153	155	156	155	
5'10	153	158	160	162	161	190
5'11	157	162	164	165	164	
6'	161	166	168	169	168	202
6'1	166	171	173	174	172	
6'2	171	176	178	179	177	215
6'3	176	181	183	184	181	
6'4	181	186	188	190	187	227

CARDIOVASCULAR RISK FACTORS

About half of all Americans eventually develop serious illnesses of the heart and blood vessels. In an average day more than 1,400 die as the result of heart attacks.

The chance of developing some form of cardiovascular disease depends partly on factors we cannot control: our age, sex and hereditary background. There are, however, several areas in which we can modify our behavior and thus improve our chances considerably.

Here are the important risk factors and some means of dealing with them:

Cigarette smoking: Stop.

High blood pressure: Have your blood pressure checked regularly by a physician. Sometimes blood pressure can be lowered by changes in diet, weight, exercise, and general lifestyle, or it may require drug therapy.

High blood cholesterol: Reduce the intake of foods high in saturated fat and cholesterol. Drug therapy may be necessary.

Diabetes: Diabetes must be treated meticulously, under the care of a physician.

Obesity: This seems to be an independent risk factor; it means that, other things being equal, overweight by itself probably poses a threat to the cardiovascular system. In any event, obesity contributes to the development of high blood pressure and invites a sedentary lifestyle, both of which are harmful.

Sedentary lifestyle: Exercise is important for the maintenance of cardiovascular health. Aside from its direct effect on the heart and blood vessels, physical activity increases the good cholesterol

(HDL) and helps to reduce stress, obesity, and high blood pressure—all of which affect risk.

Chronic unresolved stress: Stress is hard to define, because it is often an individual perception; one person's stress may be another person's "high." The most harmful stresses are probably imposed less by driving ambition, hard work, or perfectionism, than by feelings of frustration, helplessness, and an inability to cope with responsibilities or measure up to expectations.

COMMON ABBREVIATIONS, WEIGHTS, MEASURES, EQUIVALENTS

Abbreviations	Equivalents
kg = kilogram	1 kg = 1000 gm
gm = gram	1 gm = 1,000 mg
mg = milligram	1 mg = 1,000 mcg
mcg = microgram	
L = liter	1 L = 1000 ml or 1000 cc
ml = milliliter	
cc = cubic centimeter	1 kg = 2.2 lb
lb = pound	1 lb = 454 gm
oz = ounce	1 oz = 28.35 gm
gr = grain	1 gr = 65 mg
qt = quart	1 qt = 2 pt = about 960 ml
pt = pint	1 pt = 2 C = 480 ml
C = cup	1 C = 8 fl oz = 240 ml
fl oz = fluid ounce	1 fl oz = 30 ml
tbs = tablespoon	1 tbs = 15 ml
tsp = teaspoon	1 tsp = 4 ml (sometimes 5 ml)
IU or I.U. = international unit	

INDEX

CHARTS